T0286979

The Ultimate Guide to
Aromatherapy

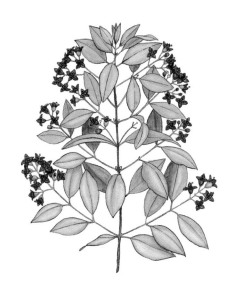

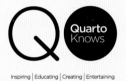

Inspiring | Educating | Creating | Entertaining

Brimming with creative inspiration, how-to projects, and useful information to enrich your everyday life, Quarto Knows is a favorite destination for those pursuing their interests and passions. Visit our site and dig deeper with our books into your area of interest: Quarto Creates, Quarto Cooks, Quarto Homes, Quarto Lives, Quarto Drives, Quarto Explores, Quarto Gifts, or Quarto Kids.

© 2020 Quarto Publishing Group USA Inc.
Text © 2020 Amy Galper and Jade Shutes

First Published in 2020 by Fair Winds Press,
an imprint of The Quarto Group,
100 Cummings Center, Suite 265-D, Beverly, MA 01915, USA.
T (978) 282-9590 F (978) 283-2742 QuartoKnows.com

Fair Winds Press titles are also available at discount for retail, wholesale, promotional, and bulk purchase. For details, contact the Special Sales Manager by email at specialsales@quarto.com or by mail at The Quarto Group, Attn: Special Sales Manager, 100 Cummings Center, Suite 265-D, Beverly, MA 01915, USA.

24 23 22 21 20   1 2 3 4 5

ISBN: 978-1-63159-897-5
Digital edition published in 2020
eISBN: 978-1-63159-898-2

Library of Congress Cataloging-in-Publication Data

Names: Galper, Amy, author. | Shutes, Jade, author.
Title: The ultimate guide to aromatherapy : an illustrated guide to blending essential oils and crafting remedies for body, mind, and spirit / Amy Galper and Jade Shutes.
Description: Beverely, MA : Fair Winds Press, 2020. | Includes bibliographical references and index. | Summary: "The Ultimate Guide to Aromatherapy is a comprehensive guide to using aromatherapy and essential oils for healing written by the co-founders of the New York Institute of Aromatic Studies"—Provided by publisher.
Identifiers: LCCN 2020012697 | ISBN 9781631598975 (trade paperback) | ISBN 9781631598982 (ebook)
Subjects: LCSH: Aromatherapy. | Essences and essential oils—Therepeutic use.
Classification: LCC RM666.A68 G35 2020 | DDC 615.3/219—dc23
LC record available at https://lccn.loc.gov/2020012697

Design and page layout: Laura Shaw Design, Inc.
Illustration: Abby Diamond /@Finchfight
Printed in China

The Ultimate Guide to
Aromatherapy

AN ILLUSTRATED GUIDE TO BLENDING ESSENTIAL OILS AND CRAFTING REMEDIES FOR BODY, MIND, AND SPIRIT

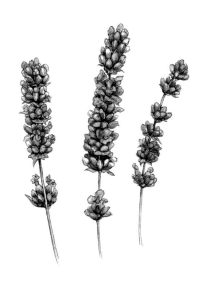

Jade Shutes & Amy Galper

WITH AMY ANTHONY, AMANDINE PETER, AND ELISABETH VLASIC

FAIR WINDS

CONTENTS

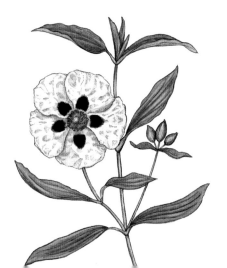

ESSENTIAL OILS

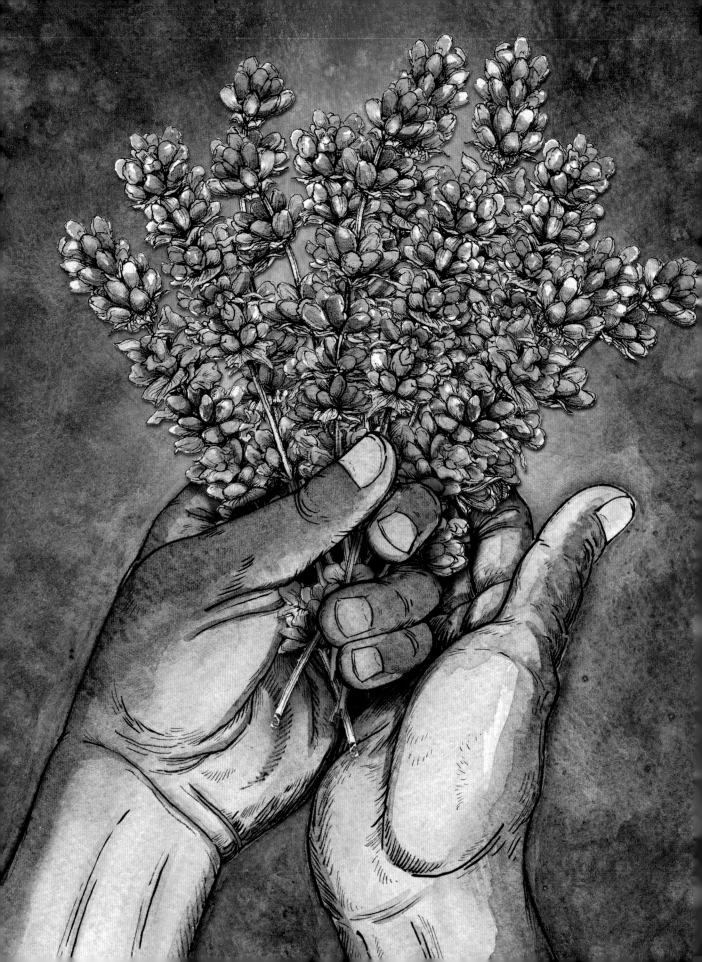

INTRODUCTION

Everyone is talking about essential oils these days. You can find ample information on them from a variety of media sources that explore their roles in herbal medicine, mindfulness, natural body care, functional medicine, and the practice of Ayurveda and Chinese medicine. But the real challenge is trusting the information you find. Who is writing it? What's their experience?

We've been around a long time, and we have garnered respect from scholars and thought leaders in the field of aromatherapy and beyond. Our students come from around the world. They find us because they want an honest, scholarly, innovative, fun, and balanced approach to learning how to use these remarkable materials.

Our approach is simple: We first celebrate the joy and beauty of the aromas of essential oils. That initial profound connection opens our minds and our hearts to the power (and science) of their medicine. We invite everyone who smells an essential oil to join our mission to connect with our sense of smell and observe how olfaction impacts our well-being and our relationships with plants and with our world.

We love essential oils. This book is our opportunity to share our passion, experience, and knowledge about aromatic plants and their power to impact our lives. Welcome to expanding your journey and deepening your understanding of essential oils!

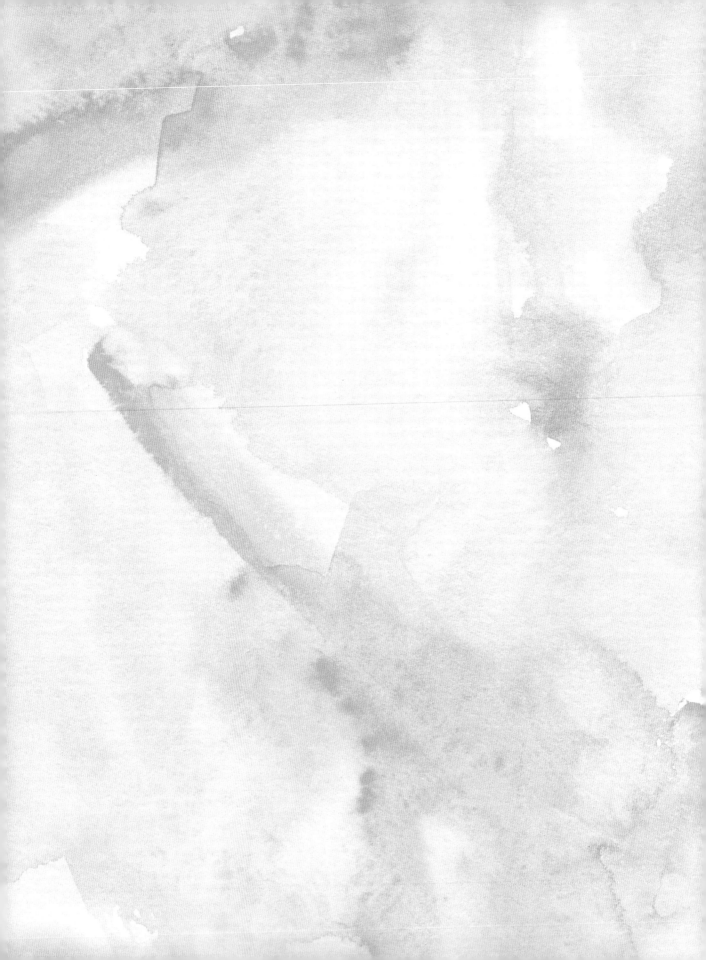

PART I

About Aromatherapy

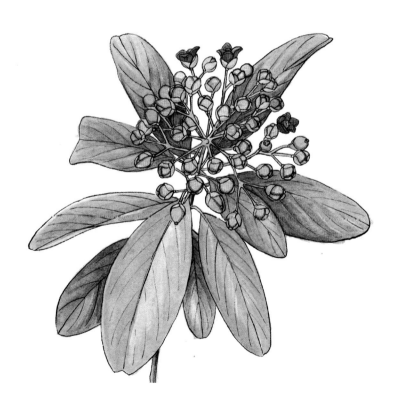

CHAPTER ONE

THE NEW AROMATHERAPY

WHAT IS AROMATHERAPY? The quick and simple answer—aromatherapy is the study and application of essential oils. It can also be referred to as Essential Oil Therapy, and that's how we like to think of it. Essential Oil Therapy (i.e., aromatherapy) encompasses the holistic application and use of essential oils to support the health and well-being of the individual. We'll use both terms in this book.

But if we dig deeper, its true and genuine definition is still a little murky. It's often misunderstood and undervalued, possibly due to its commercial exploitation, especially in the United States. Think of all the diffusers saturating the market these days, and the thousands of articles and Internet posts touting the magical powers of essential oils. (That's actually one of the reasons we like calling it Essential Oil Therapy.) And yet, despite the lack of clarity and complexity in its definition, aromatherapy continues to be one of the fastest growing complementary healthcare modalities of the 21st century.

Before we start carving out our approach to Essential Oil Therapy, let's quickly review the history of the human use of aromatic plants. Understanding it can provide great insight into how we redefine it for the 21st century.

Although humans have been using aromatic plants for thousands of years, aromatherapy as we know it today is a relatively young practice in comparison. Throughout this book you will be introduced to the remarkably dynamic and diverse ways in which essential oils can be used: house-cleaning products, therapeutic inhalers, diffuser blends, body care products to nourish and support the health of skin, and medicinal products that support the body's own innate healing processes.

A LITTLE HISTORY

Our use of medicinal and aromatic plants is ancient. Many of the ways our ancestors used aromatics are similar to the ways in which we use them today. They date back to the origins of humans, when aromatic plant material was first placed onto a fire. Our sense of smell was more attuned back then, and primitive humans may have found the aromas powerfully affecting them in many ways.

Eventually, through their intuition and observations, people were motivated to start writing down their experiences with plants. We can find written records dating as far back as 5,000 years. Cultures in India, Egypt, and China, for example, have rich histories and evidence of using medicinal and aromatic plants. Plants collected for their aroma and extracts were used for medicine, food preservation, religious ceremonies, and embalming the dead.

During the Middle Ages aromatics were used for defense against the bubonic plague. Doctors would use a variety of aromatic herbs and spices stuffed in

Market research studies, conducted by Grand View Research in April 2019 and Market Reports World in September 2019, report that the global aromatherapy market size was valued at USD $1.3 billion in 2018 and is projected to witness a 10.4 percent CAGR (compound annual growth rate) over the forecast period ending in 2025. Rising awareness about therapeutic uses of essential oils is anticipated to drive the growth. Specifically, Grand View's *Aromatherapy Market Size Analysis* reports that revenues are expected to reach $2.35 billion by 2025.

a mask to protect themselves from infection. It has been speculated that through their use of aromatics, perfumers and glove makers (those who made gloves would imbue the gloves with aromatics) were immune to the plague due to the aromatics they used in their respective crafts.

By the 18th century, the use of essential oils was much more widespread. Research on their medicinal properties captivated the curiosity of physicians and druggists, who were the early precursors to modern pharmacists. And in the 19th century, published studies showing the antibacterial and antifungal properties of many essential oils became more accessible.

Let's take a brief look at how the word *Aromatherapy* came into the modern lexicon. It was René-Maurice Gattefossé, perfumer and chemist, who coined the term in 1937. Probably the most important thing to remember about Gattefossé and his impact on what eventually grew into the modern practice of aromatherapy is that he clearly meant to distinguish the medicinal application of essential oils from their perfumery applications.

As a perfumer, he had a great love and passion for the aromas of essential oils, but by 1918 he grew more fascinated with their application for medicinal purposes.

Fast Forward 100 Years

Today our definition of aromatherapy is much more nuanced. We recognize and implement the dual effect essential oils have on the body and the mind.

This modern perspective was mostly born from the work of visionary Marguerite Maury (1895–1968), a traditionally trained nurse from Vienna who had a passion for exploring mind and body practices, such as acupuncture, yoga, and meditation.

Her fascination with and great love of aromatics compelled her to explore how best to apply essential oils to achieve a notable and identifiable connection between the mind and body. From this, she pioneered the practice of applying essential oils topically and observing their psychological and physiological benefits.

If we want to celebrate and advocate a new paradigm that integrates the holistic nature of essential oils into 21st century concepts of health and well-being, it's key for us to understand her work and her influential contributions.

Maury's work helped build the foundational and philosophical framework for the modern practice of holistic aromatherapy:

- **Integration of massage and aromatherapy.** A strong advocate of massage to maintain good health, Maury saw it as an opportunity to deliver essential oils to the body.

- **The importance of a holistic approach.** Health must be maintained through the balance of diet, exercise, emotional support, and spiritual support.

- **The importance of the individual.** Like Maury, we emphasize the value of creating aromatic remedies based upon the individual's needs and health concerns.

- **Recognition of the dual effect of essential oils.** Essential oils, when applied to the skin, not only have a physiological effect, but also a corresponding psychological effect.

WHAT IT MEANS TO BE HEALTHY IN THE 21ST CENTURY

To really understand how using essential oils can improve our health and well-being, we must first rethink what it means to be healthy.

Orthodox medicine focuses primarily on treating symptoms and diseases, and often doesn't pay much attention to what may be causing the problems. This approach leaves us believing that to feel healthy, we have to be symptom-free. But is this really what being healthy means?

Let's consider another option. What if we let go of this notion that feeling good and living well are the result of not having any physical or emotional symptoms? Instead we could start thinking about our health, and our ability to heal, as finding balance in our lives.

Today, Essential Oil Therapy is considered a Holistic Health Modality. It focuses on healing the patient by addressing the nature of the disease within the context of the whole person, including diet, lifestyle, exercise, stress levels, and anything else that may be contributing to or potentially causing the disease or imbalance. The goal is to attain balance—physically, mentally, emotionally, socially, and spiritually. And thanks to Maury, we are inspired to look at the uniqueness of each individual and appreciate each person's set of criteria and challenges.

Where aromatherapy shines as practice is in supporting us when we are off balance. It's not intended to create whole health or wellness, or to cure or heal us from disease. Of course, we know that using essential oils for acute conditions, such as injuries, pain, or infections, can have great results that have been well documented. But the true nature and power of Essential Oil Therapy is to help our minds and bodies find their way back to balance.

Let's take a look at our diagram (opposite). Here we can see that our goal, illustrated in the center, is to find what we call Radiant Health. But affecting the stability of this constantly moving center are all the factors we are faced with every day, which threaten to throw us off our game and prevent us from finding that sense of place.

We've all had those days, or weeks, when we don't sleep well, we are experiencing grief or loss, or we've been too busy to exercise or spend time outside in nature. When that happens, our center gets thrown off, and we begin to feel symptoms such as sore muscles, digestive issues, and anxiety. And that's the moment we should be reaching for essential oils. By doing so, we can potentially prevent the imbalances from escalating into more serious health problems.

This book will show you how using essential oils can help you do this. We will explain the properties of the essential oils and share recipes and best practices for how to apply them. We will do this guided by our intention to make their use accessible—so you, too, can find your place of balance.

OUR PREFERRED METHOD: THE NEW AROMATHERAPY

We've been teaching about essential oils since the early 1990s. After all these years and thousands of students, we've become even more committed to and passionate about the holistic nature of essential

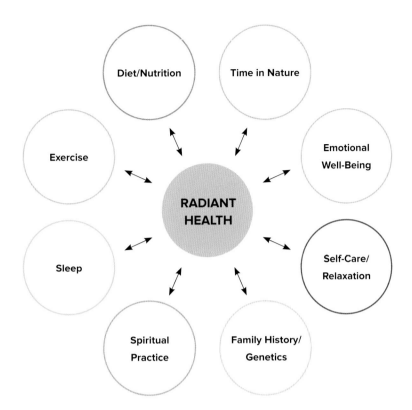

oils and their power to make profound changes in our lives. Smelling and working with them for all these years has shown us how profoundly they can impact our experience of our world.

As educators and advocates, we are dedicated to sharing our knowledge and experience. We want our students to understand our perspective so that they can use essential oils to live more consciously. To make our concepts more accessible, we have distilled our unique approach into a simple method. As you read this book, you will discover our framework, core principles, and practice echoed throughout each chapter.

This pioneering, balanced, innovative, and progressive approach teaches the basic concepts of aromatherapy in order to help people live more consciously, by using the profound holistic nature of

essential oils as the core catalyst to inspire change. It provides a modern, heart-centered philosophical framework to guide teachers, students, and laypeople to live healthier and inspired lives.

The Framework: Shifting the Paradigm

The philosophical foundation of this method is built upon a framework focused on supporting the body versus treating disease. Our method informs how we utilize essential oils to:

- Stimulate and support the body's innate ability to heal.
- Encompass the whole (individual) person.
- Address the underlying cause of a disease or imbalance.

ACUTE INTERVENTION
Followed by building terrain and resiliency.

SYMPTOM RELIEF
Relieve acute pain; reduce anxiety.

VIS MEDICATRIX NATURAE
Stimulate and support self-healing.

NOURISHMENT
Feed the "self," mind/body, etc. Includes massage, spa, esthetics (facials), reflexology.

TERRAIN
Includes diet/whole foods, lifestyle, exercise, herbs, and essential oils, hydrosols, aromatherapy, gardening, soil, nutritional supplements, community, and time in nature.

HEART

- Consider the aroma therapist as a teacher.
- Focus on prevention.
- Live by the Hippocratic code to First Do No Harm.

The Core Principles

Keep these important principles in mind as you build your knowledge and practice:

- Knowledge is Art (intuition) + Science (facts).
- Aromatherapy is the quintessential expression of holistic healthcare, meaning it encompasses physical, emotional, and at times, spiritual health and wellness.
- Know the Person, rather than the Disease.
- Utilize intention and mindfulness.
- Understand the significance of relationships
  ▷ Client and practitioner
  ▷ Practitioner and oils
  ▷ Boundaries, personal and professional
  ▷ To Nature (plants)
  ▷ To Self

The Core Practice

Our method is practically applied via three core methodologies. These methodologies offer specific guidelines for blending essential oils and revolutionizing the way in which practitioners, teachers, and natural beauty entrepreneurs approach formulation, through the lens of wellness and healing.

1. Blending: Our approach to formulating.
2. Consultation: Our comprehensive approach to clinical practice.
3. Plant Relationship(s): Our belief in the power of our relationship with nature to heal and transform.

CHAPTER TWO

AROMATIC PLANTS TO ESSENTIAL OILS

ESSENTIAL OILS are highly concentrated aromatic extracts that are distilled or expressed from a variety of plant material, including flowers, flowering tops, fruits/zests, grasses, leaves, needles and twigs, resins, roots, seeds, and woods.

Through the process of converting energy from the sun (photosynthesis), plants produce not only the food they need to survive but a host of secondary plant chemicals to support their health and survival. Some of these secondary chemicals are what make up essential oils.

Technically, while in the plant, essential oils are actually a collection of many volatile chemicals (components) stored within the plant. These volatile components are responsible for the aroma and part of the taste of many medicinal plants. While in the plant, they are constantly changing their composition, helping the plant to adapt to an ever-changing internal and external environment.

WHY DO PLANTS PRODUCE ESSENTIAL OILS?

Plants produce aromatic components to:

- **Attract insects:** A variety of insects, from bees to butterflies, are attracted to flowering plants due to their aroma, color, or physical appearance. Scent is one of the most ancient and common ways plants can attract pollinators for the purpose of reproduction.

- **Repel competition:** Aromatic plants can send out volatile chemical messages to other plants to prevent them from growing and competing for limited resources within their area or zone.

- **Protect against predators:** Plants can release a complex mixture of volatile oils, or terpenes, to deter insects and other animals from approaching them.

- **Defend and protect:** Plants can produce an array of antimicrobial, antifungal, and antibacterial agents to protect themselves from a wide range of organisms that may threaten their survival.

WHERE DO PLANTS STORE ESSENTIAL OILS?

Plants store volatile components either in external secretory structures found on the surface of the plant or in internal secretory structures found inside a part or parts of the plant.

For plants that have external secretory structures, all you have to do is rub your hand or fingers on the leaf and its aroma is imparted to your skin. But for plants with internal secretory structures, you will need to break open the leaf, cut into the root, or press the peel to release the essential oil.

- **Plants with external secretory structures** include basil, lavender, sweet marjoram, melissa (lemon balm), oregano, peppermint, rosemary, and spearmint.

- **Plants with internal secretory structures** include citrus fruits, eucalyptus, frankincense, angelica, and most other essential oils.

EXTRACTING ESSENTIAL OILS

The two main processes used to extract essential oils are distillation and expression. Other processes, such as enfleurage and solvent extraction, produce aromatic products called *absolutes*. The CO_2 extraction process produces CO_2 extracts.

Distillation: An Alchemical Process

Distillation has been practiced throughout history. In the early Middle Ages, a crude form of distillation was used primarily to prepare floral waters or distilled aromatic waters. These appear to have been used in perfumery, as digestive tonics, in cooking, and for trading.

During distillation, the plant material is placed upon a grid inside a still. Then the still is sealed and

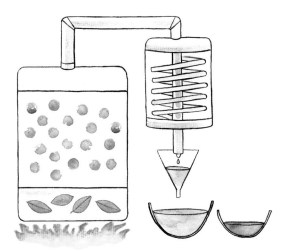

steam or a combination of water and steam slowly breaks through the plant material to remove its volatile components. These volatile components rise upward through a connecting pipe that leads them into a condenser. The condenser cools the rising vapor back into liquid form. The liquid is then collected in a container below the condenser. Because water and essential oil do not mix, the essential oil is found on the surface of the water where it is siphoned off. Occasionally an essential oil such as clove is heavier than water and is found on the bottom.[1]

Expression

Expression, also called cold pressing or *ècuelle à piquer*, is a method of extraction specific to citrus essential oils such as tangerine, lemon, bergamot, sweet orange, and lime.

Expressed citrus oils are produced by mechanical separation (cold pressing) of the oil from the peels of the fruits. Expressed citrus oils offer the advantage of cold process, which results in an aroma identical to fresh citrus peels.

What is the difference between expressed and distilled citrus essential oils? Some aromatherapy companies sell both versions from the same species. The main differences between distilled and expressed citrus essential oils have to do with their toxicity, volatility, and aroma. Distilled citrus oils tend to deteriorate more quickly and are considerably more unstable than the expressed oils. (See page 23 for more on the safety concerns for different types of citrus extractions.)

Solvent Extraction

Not all aromatic plant material can be distilled or expressed, as it may be too fragile to hold up to the distillation process. Plants such as jasmine, tuberose, carnation, gardenia, jonquil, violet leaf, narcissus, mimosa, and other delicate flowers are extracted using solvent extraction.

Solvent extraction is the use of solvents, such as petroleum ether, methanol, ethanol, or hexane, to extract the aromatic lipophilic (fat soluble) material from the plant. The solvent will also pull out the chlorophyll and other plant tissue, resulting in a highly colored or thick/viscous extract. After some processing, the final product is known as an *absolute*.

Absolutes are highly concentrated aromatic substances that will most often resemble the natural aroma of the plant and are normally more colored and viscous than essential oils. Absolutes are used extensively in the botanical perfume and cosmetics industry.

CO_2 Hypercritical Extraction

Hypercritical carbon dioxide (CO_2) extraction produces CO_2 extracts that are becoming increasingly popular. How does CO_2 work? Basically, when carbon dioxide is under pressure, it will turn from a gas into a liquid. This liquid can then be used as an inert liquid solvent able to diffuse throughout the plant material, thus extracting various components from the plant. Substances that can be extracted include essential oil components, waxes, pigments, lipids, and resins.

WHAT TO LOOK FOR WHEN PURCHASING CO_2 EXTRACTS

CO_2 is available as total extracts and select extracts.

Total extracts contain all the possible CO_2-extracted components from the plant material, which can make them quite thick and a bit challenging to work with. The essential oil component content can vary between 3 percent and 50 percent of the total extract, with the remaining extract being composed of waxes, lipids, and the like, depending on the plant material. Warming thick CO_2 extracts helps make them easier to use. Because total extracts contain the lipid components, there are some incredible CO_2 extracts that act more like carriers or herbal oils than essential oils. Examples of these types of total CO_2 extracts include calendula CO_2 (see page 153, arnica CO_2, rosehip CO_2, and sea buckthorn CO_2).

Select extracts contain mostly the essential oil components, which can make up 35 percent to 95 percent of the extract. Select extracts are not viscous like total extracts and hence are easier to use.

Select CO_2 extracts contain many of the same constituents as their essential oil counterparts, although they may also contain some components not found in essential oils. For instance, the essential oil of ginger (*Zingiber officinale*) does not contain the bitter principles (shogaol, gingerols), but the CO_2 extract does. Select CO_2 extracts are known for their strong similarity in aroma to the actual plant aroma versus the essential oil, which can smell slightly different from the actual plant.

NOTE: Due to the potential of pesticide residue in CO_2 extracts, we recommend organic CO_2 extracts only.

ESSENTIAL OIL CHEMISTRY

An individual essential oil can be made up of more than 200 individual components, many at less than 0.1 percent of the final mixture. These chemical components are categorized into families. Specifically, essential oils contain simple terpenes in the form of monoterpenes and sesquiterpenes, and more complex terpenoids in the form of alcohols, phenols, phenylpropanoids, esters, aldehydes, ketones, oxides, sesquiterpene lactones, and furano-coumarins. Each chemical family contains unique chemical components that not only make up the whole essential oil, but also support its therapeutic activity, and at times are the reason for an oil's potential toxicity.

Chemical Families in Essential Oils

This chart reviews the chemical families in oils, including examples of components along with general therapeutics for that family. The essential oils listed are examples of ones rich in that family of chemicals.

FAMILY	GENERAL THERAPEUTICS	ESSENTIAL OILS
Monoterpenes d-limonene, myrcene, α-pinene, β-pinene, β-ocimene, α-terpinene, α-phellandrene, camphene, (-)-car-3-ene	• Antimicrobial • Antioxidant • Drying/dehydrating effect • Energizing/uplifting	Citrus essential oils (e.g., Bergamot, Sweet Orange) Cypress Juniper Berry Pine
Sesquiterpenes β-bisabolene, chamazulene, α-cedrene, aromadendrene, germacrene D, β-cadinene, ar-curcumene, β-elemene, α-caryophyllene, β-sesquiphellandrene	• Powerful anti-inflammatory • Antispasmodic • Moderate antimicrobials • Calming and soothing to the nervous system • Anti-allergic	German Chamomile Copaiba Tansy Turmeric
Monoterpene Alcohols borneol, lavandulol, nerol, citronellol, linalool, terpinen-4-ol, geraniol, menthol, α-terpineol	• Antimicrobial (antibacterial, antifungal, antiviral) • Anti-inflammatory • Antioxidant • Antispasmodic • Mild and well tolerated by the skin • Sedative	Bergamot Coriander Seed Geranium Sweet Marjoram Lavender
Sesquiterpene Alcohols α-bisabolol, daucol, α-santalol, carotol, farnesol, β-santalol, cedrol, patchoulol, zingiberol	• Anti-inflammatory • Antimicrobial • Antifungal • Calming and soothing (nervous system, endocrine system, and emotions) • Most have strong affinity with the skin	Carrot Seed Clary Sage German Chamomile Patchouli Sandalwood

$\rightarrow$

FAMILY	GENERAL THERAPEUTICS	ESSENTIAL OILS
Esters bornyl acetate, methyl salicylate, geranyl acetate, linalyl acetate, isobutyl angelate, thymol acetate, benzyl acetate	• Anti-inflammatory • Antispasmodic • Direct effect on the central nervous system (CNS): Relaxing and balancing • Release muscular and nervous tension • Soothing to dermal inflammation	Bergamot Cape Chamomile Clary Sage Inula Petitgrain
Aldehydes	• Antibacterial • Antifungal • Antiviral • Anti-inflammatory • Anxiolytic • Sedative • Potential skin irritants	Citronella Eucalyptus citriodora Lemongrass Melissa May Chang (Litsea cubeba)
Ketones	• Mucolytic • Promote skin and tissue regeneration • Wound healing agent • Anti-inflammatory	Turmeric Pennyroyal Spearmint Dill Caraway
Phenols thymol, carvacrol, eugenol	• Analgesic • Anti-inflammatory • Antibacterial • Antifungal • Airborne antimicrobial • Warming	Clove Bud Thyme ct. thymol Oregano Winter Savory Cinnamon Leaf
Phenylpropanoids cis-anethole, trans-anethole, methyl chavicol syn. estragole, safrole, cinnamaldehyde, methyl eugenol	• Analgesic • Antimicrobial • Antifungal • Anti-inflammatory • Antispasmodic • Stress modulating • Digestive	Anise Basil Cinnamon Bark Fennel Sassafras
Oxides/Ethers specifically: 1,8 cineole, also known as eucalyptol	• Analgesic • Anti-inflammatory • Antiviral (respiratory) • Antibacterial (respiratory) • Powerful expectorant • Decongestant (respiratory) • Mucolytic • Immunomodulatory	Eucalyptus Niaouli Tea Tree Bay Laurel Rosemary ct. cineole

Two other chemical families are furanocoumarins and sesquiterpene lactones. Furanocoumarins are typically found in very low concentrations. However, bergapten, the most common furanocoumarin, is responsible for the photosensitizing action of bergamot and other citrus essential oils. Sesquiterpene lactones are found in the essential oils of inula (as small amounts of alantolactone and isolantolactone) and catnip, which contains various isomers of nepetalactone as its major components.

ESSENTIAL OIL SAFETY

With so much emphasis these days on safety and essential oils, it seems that the challenge isn't really about "more safety" but rather how shall we relate to it? How shall we interpret it so that it makes sense in our practice or general use of essential oils? And how shall we find balance within the extremes that appear on social media?

Our philosophy is that essential oils are safe. It seems simple enough, right? And yet, there are four important caveats:

1. *Essential oils are safe* when selected appropriately for the individual or purpose of the product.

2. *Essential oils are safe* when the appropriate method of application (body oil, steam inhalation, baths, etc.) is chosen correctly for the individual or purpose of the product.

3. *Essential oils are safe* when the correct dilution of the essential oil is used.

4. *Essential oils are safe* when the individual has the appropriate level of knowledge and experience with each essential oil they are using.

Essential oils are powerful. They speak on multiple levels (physiologically and emotionally) to the human organism and are capable of wildly diverse yet complementary therapeutic actions

"If we recognize essential oils fundamentally as familiar allies rather than alien foes, we can then assume the wider perspective of them being inherently safe rather than unsafe."

—PETER HOLMES,
Aromatica Volume 1: Principles and Profiles

(antispasmodic, anti-inflammatory, etc.). Humans co-evolved with aromatic and medicinal plants, which have been our allies as food, as shelter, in magic or ritual, as aromas and olfactory delight, and as medicine. We have a symbiotic relationship. But, like in all relationships, we must cultivate our inherent respect for their power and their potency and use them accordingly.[2]

A Positive Approach: Essential Oil Safety

In his book *Aromatica*, Peter Holmes shares the idea of creating a positive context for essential oil safety. Inspired by his writing, we have adopted and modified his model to create three categories of essential oils for home use as well as for the aromatherapist.

We hope, like Peter Holmes, to inspire a new way of viewing and relating to the safety of essential oils—one through the lens of the *knowledgeable, responsible, reflective,* and *empowered* aromatherapist and essential oil therapist. There are three categories of essential oils.

Category 1: Mild Essential Oils

This category includes most essential oils commonly used at home and in practice. The essential oils in this category are considered to be generally safe and without risk of toxicity or accumulation, even when used over an extended period of time. Specific essential oils in this group may also have unique safety information (e.g., photosensitizer, irritant).

Mild essential oils

Most essential oils, including Cape Chamomile, Cardamom, Carrot Seed, Cedarwood, Roman Chamomile, German Chamomile, Citrus Oils, Cilantro, Clary Sage, Cypress, Fennel, Fir, Frankincense, Geranium, Ginger, Lavender, Lavandin, Melissa, Pine, Rose, Saro, Tea Tree.

Category 2: Strong Essential Oils

This group of essential oils presents some potential or risk of toxic accumulation of certain components, regardless of method of application. The essential oils below should be used with caution. The main concern is for neurotoxicity (negative impact on the nervous system). Be cautious with dermal applications, be sure to dilute them, and avoid daily long-term application (>10–30 days).

Essential oils in this category are contraindicated (not appropriate for use) during pregnancy or while breastfeeding.

Strong essential oils

- Sage (*Salvia officinalis*), α-thujone, β-thujone and camphor

- Rosemary ct. verbenone (*Rosmarinus officinalis*), verbenone

- Hyssop ct. pinocamphone (*Hyssopus officinalis*), pinocamphone

- Rosemary ct. camphor (*Rosmarinus officinalis*), camphor[3]

"Ingesting 3 drops of any of these oils constitutes an excessive dose with potentially serious toxicity."

—KURT SCHNAUBELT,
The Healing Intelligence of Essential Oils

Category 3: Powerful Essential Oils

Essential oils in this group can cause acute poisoning regardless of route of administration. The oral use of these essential oils should be avoided due to potential for liver and nervous system toxicity. These oils are best avoided unless you have received proper education and training on their use and application.

Powerful essential oils with potential for acute toxicity

- Mugwort (*Artemisia vulgaris*), thujone

- Sage (*Salvia officinalis*), thujone

- *Hyssopus officinalis* NOT *Hyssopus officinalis* var. *decumbens*

- *Lavandula stoechas,* thujone

- Wormwood (*Artemisia absinthium*), thujone

- Cedar leaf (*Thuja occidentalis*), thujone

- Pennyroyal (*Mentha pulegium*), pulegone[4]

OTHER SAFETY ISSUES

Along with the categories above, it is important to also know any specific safety concerns for each individual essential oil you have. And because so many aromatherapy products are applied to the skin, be aware of potential skin reactions. The three main skin reactions are irritation, sensitization, and photosensitization.

Irritation

Irritation is when a substance applied to the skin produces an immediate irritating effect. The appearance of the skin may be blotchy and red, and it may be painful or feel like it is burning. The severity of the reaction will depend on the concentration (dilution) and the specific essential oil applied. Avoid using undiluted dermal irritants on the skin, and avoid using even diluted oils on inflamed, open, or damaged skin.

Skin irritating essential oils include cinnamon bark, citronella, clove bud, lemongrass, oregano, thyme ct. thymol, winter savory.

Sensitization

Sensitization is either an immediate or, more commonly, a delayed allergic response that involves the immune system. Cinnamon bark (and to some extent, the leaf) and clove bud are good examples of essential oils that can cause both immediate and delayed sensitization responses. Delayed sensitization means that although there may be no reaction upon the first or even after several applications, eventually an inflammatory reaction occurs.

What does it look like on the skin? There will be a red rash or darker area of the skin (in darker color skin), reflecting damage caused by substances such as histamine released in the dermis due to an immune response.[5]

The problem with sensitization is that once it occurs with a specific essential oil, the individual is most likely going to be sensitive to it for many years and perhaps for the remainder of his or her life. The best way to prevent sensitization is to avoid applying known dermal sensitizers to the skin.

Skin sensitizers include cinnamon bark; oxidized oils of pine, fir, and other conifers; all citrus essential oils.

Photosensitization

Photosensitization is a reaction to a substance applied to the skin that occurs only in the presence of UV light in the UVA range. Photosensitizing essential oils will cause burning or skin pigmentation changes, such as tanning, upon exposure to sun or similar light (ultraviolet rays). Reactions can range from a mild color change to deep weeping burns. *Do not use or recommend the use of photosensitizing essential oils prior to going into a tanning booth or out into the sun for at least 12 hours after application.*

Certain drugs, such as tetracycline, increase the photosensitivity of the skin, thus increasing the harmful effects of photosensitizing essential oils under the necessary conditions.

Photosensitizing essential oils include angelica root, bergamot, expressed lemon, expressed lime, and expressed bitter orange. Distilled or expressed grapefruit has a low risk for photosensitization.

These citrus oils are not photosensitizing: distilled lemon, distilled lime, mandarin, bergamot FCF, sweet orange, yuzu (distilled or expressed).

PURCHASING ESSENTIAL OILS

Before we dive into individual essential oils, let's review what you want to know when purchasing them. To begin, you will want to be sure to have the following information:

- **Common name**

- **Latin name** (exact genus and species): Note that some essential oil plants, such as lavender, have different species.

- **Part of the plant processed:** Some plants produce essential oils from different parts, such as the root or the seed. It is important to know what part of the plant was used to distill the essential oil.

- **Type of extraction:** (distillation, expression, CO_2, or solvent extraction)

- **How it was grown:** (organic, wild-crafted, traditional, etc.)

- **Chemotype** (when relevant)

- **Country of origin**

- **Sustainability:** With growing concern for overharvesting and changes in weather patterns, it is the responsibility of those using essential oils to be sure they have been harvested from a sustainable source.

Of equal importance to all of the above criteria is your own sensory assessment. Naturally, when it comes to essential oils, this means first and foremost your sense of smell. However, the ability to smell (or sense) the "quality" or "wholeness" of an essential oil requires some practice and lots of patience.

Here's how to powerfully utilize your sense of smell for determining the quality of essential oils. Each of these steps takes time, patience, consciousness, and willingness.

"The quality and authenticity of the essential oils we utilize are the very heart and foundation of aromatherapy."

—JADE SHUTES

1. Strengthen your sense of smell

The sense of smell, in our experience, is like a muscle. The more you use it and become aware of it, the stronger it becomes. To exercise your sense of smell, simply become conscious of the various aromas in your environment or in places you go. Spend 2 to 4 weeks simply observing, becoming aware of the different aromas that waft under your nose each day.

2. Strengthen your relationship with aromatic plants

Even though most of us will never go to Madagascar or Costa Rica to smell ylang ylang as it lingers on the tree, there are still many aromatic plants you may have access to in a variety of settings.

We recommend spending time with a wide variety of aromatic plants, if and when possible. Obviously, the spring and summer months (particularly late spring and summer, when the essential oil content is higher) are the best times to explore aromatic plants. Get started in your own garden or at an arboretum, a garden center, an herb farm, or even in nature. This relationship with aromatic plants is key in being able to appropriately utilize your sense of smell when it comes to the quality and wholeness of essential oils.

Strengthening our relationship with aromatic plants strengthens our relationship with the essential oils they give forth. It provides us with a much wider olfactory palate and empowers our sense of smell in better perceiving a quality essential oil from one of inferior quality.

3. Compare and contrast essential oils

Now let's talk about using your sense of smell with actual essential oils. To be able to understand and interpret the differences between qualities of essential oils, one must spend time with and be exposed to different qualities (and therefore, different "brands"). Spend time with the essential oils you get from different companies or find in different stores, as this expands your olfactory palette.

THE QUALITIES OF ESSENTIAL OILS

Essential oils display a set of general physical characteristics that give them their identity.

- Essential oils are highly concentrated, which means they are powerful substances. This is one of the reasons they are diluted into a carrier for application to the skin. Their strength also means a little goes a long way.

- Essential oils are highly complex chemical substances often containing hundreds of unique components. This chemistry is the backbone of the wide range of therapeutic activity essential oils have to offer.

- Essential oils have volatility, which means they can turn from liquid to vapor. Some essential oils, such as citrus oils, are more volatile than others, such as vetiver. This leads us to the next quality.

- Essential oils are light and not greasy. The name *essential oil* can be deceptive. Essential oils are not vegetable or fatty oils; rather they are light, volatile substances that are referred to as "oils." They have a consistency more like water (although they are insoluble in water) than oil and lack the oily texture of vegetable oils (except for viscous essential oils, such as sandalwood, vetiver, and myrrh).

**WHAT IS THE SHELF LIFE
OF AN ESSENTIAL OIL?**

* *For monoterpene-rich essential oils* such as citrus oils, conifers (pine, spruce, hemlock), frankincense, lemongrass, neroli, and tea tree: 1 to 2 years

* *For all other essential oils:* 2 to 3 years

* *For viscous essential oils* such as vetiver, patchouli, and sandalwood: 4 to 8+ years

ESSENTIAL OIL STORAGE TIPS

* Store essential oils in amber, black, or blue glass bottles to protect them from the potentially damaging effects of light.

* Make sure bottles have an orifice reducer, which helps prevent oxygen from aging the essential oils and also helps control the flow of drops.

* Keep essential oils away from light and heat and in a cool place or room to enhance their shelf life and keep their vitality.

- Essential oils are mostly clear to light yellow in color. There are a few blue oils, such as German chamomile, tansy, and yarrow. Patchouli can be dark brown, while inula has a magnificent emerald green color.

- Essential oils are attracted to and soluble in fatty substances such as vegetable oils (carrier oils), herbal oils, and unscented creams and lotions.

- Some essential oils are thick or viscous. Vetiver is a key example of a viscous essential oil. Unlike a citrus essential oil, which flows out of the bottle, vetiver flows slowly out of the bottle due to its thickness (viscosity). Viscous essential oils are less volatile and tend to have a heavier aroma.

PART II

Pathways into the Body

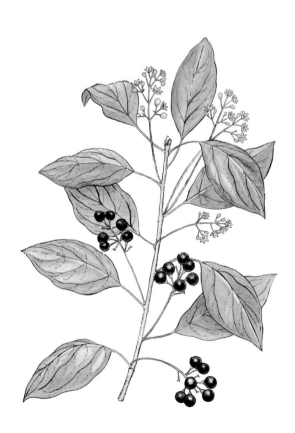

CHAPTER THREE

AROMATHERAPY AND THE SKIN

EVERYTHING THAT TOUCHES the skin has an effect not only on the skin itself but potentially on the entire physical body. Applying essential oils to the skin—in a suitable medium—is one of the most dynamic ways to enjoy the incredible benefits they offer. Once on the skin, essential oils may support cellular rejuvenation, relieve itchiness, reduce inflammation and irritation from an insect bite, and much more, as you will discover. Through the power of essential oils and carrier bases, aromatherapy body care products support, protect, and enhance our skin's overall health and vibrancy.

Think about how many products we put on our skin daily. According to the Environmental Working Group (EWG), women apply an average of as many as 12 different products to their skin daily, while men apply an average of up to six.[6] The EWG has also raised concerns regarding some of the potential health impacts (from cancer to hormonal dysfunction) of phthalates, parabens, and other chemicals found in some personal care products.

Aromatherapy body care products, on the other hand, tend to be made from simple ingredients, most of which are plant based. All of the ingredients, when used properly, can support the skin's health and the overall health of the entire body and emotions (mind).

Aromatherapy body care products not only address skin imbalances, they also use the skin as a medium to address other imbalances such as muscular aches and pains, painful cramps during menstruation, and much more.

PATHWAYS INTO THE BODY

Essential oils have four potential pathways into the body: the skin, the sense of smell (olfaction), the respiratory system, and ingestion.[7] In this chapter, we explore the skin as a pathway for essential oils and other botanical ingredients such as carrier oils and herbal oils.

Before we dive into all the amazing benefits essential oils have for the skin specifically, let's look at products that are applied to the skin not for skin care but to address other issues or imbalances occurring in the body.

Circulatory (Cardiovascular) System

When it comes to the cardiovascular system, exercise and healthy eating are the first things to consider if a health imbalance is occurring. However, essential oils (in an appropriate carrier or base) applied to the skin can support and enhance healthy circulation and reduce the appearance of varicose veins. Gels are the preferred medium for varicose veins.

Our favorite way to support healthy circulation is to use salt scrubs, although body oils and aromatic baths can be beneficial too.

DEFINITION: BODY CARE PRODUCT

Throughout this book, when we refer to body care products, we mean a combination of essential oils with some type of base, such as a carrier oil and/or herbal oil, an unscented cream or lotion, or a gel or salve.

Digestive System

An abdominal massage oil is often indicated when working with digestive upsets such as constipation, excess gas, stomach cramps, or stress-related digestive conditions. Massaging using a carrier oil and essential oils with an affinity to the digestive system can help to relieve general constipation caused by travel, change in diet, poor diet, etc.; to relieve painful gas; or reduce and relieve stress-related digestive upsets.

Addressing dietary changes and lifestyle factors is a priority for most digestive conditions.

Musculoskeletal System

Body oils, gels, salves, and even body butters, creams, and lotions can all be used when working with muscular or joint aches and pains. Essential oils, carrier oils, or herbal oils can be selected to:

- relieve joint pain
- reduce muscular aches and pains
- relieve tension, relax muscles
- reduce muscle spasms
- speed recovery from sprains, strains, and repetitive movement injuries.

Respiratory System

The most common aromatherapy product applied to the skin for the respiratory system is a salve, although a cream or chest oil may also be used.

INTERNAL USE OF ESSENTIAL OILS

We we will be covering aromatherapy and essential oil content relevant to applying essential oils to the skin and via inhalation or diffusion (olfaction and respiratory system). Although we believe in the efficacy of utilizing essential oils internally, that topic is not covered in this book. We believe that this requires further education than what we could share in a book of this nature and length.

A respiratory salve is applied to the chest, neck, back, and under the nose (for people more than 7 years old only). The salve is beneficial for relieving congestion while supporting the entire respiratory system in recovering from common respiratory ailments such as the cold or flu. Essential oils in the salve may be used to:

- relieve congestion by supporting the elimination of excess mucus
- prevent or minimize hay fever
- relieve spasmodic coughing
- support the respiratory system and body in overcoming or recovering from respiratory infection, cold, flu, and other common respiratory ailments
- open up and expand breathing.

Reproductive System

Applying essential oils in a suitable carrier oil, cream, or lotion can be incredibly beneficial for relieving painful menstrual cramps and other imbalances associated with menstruation, perimenopause, and menopause. Essential oils applied to the skin can alleviate pain and cramps associated with menstruation and support emotional wellness.

Every aromatherapy product applied to the skin, for skin health or for another body system, will naturally have an effect on the mind and emotions. We'll be exploring how emotions affect the skin and vice versa in a moment. First, let's meet your skin!

By acquainting ourselves with how this multifunctional, amazingly dynamic, and sophisticated organ is structured and how it functions, we will not only feel more confident and at ease when choosing specific essential oils and other botanical ingredients (e.g., carrier oils) to apply topically, but we will also be able to fully understand how these botanical substances interact with our skin, are partially absorbed, and ultimately affect the ever-changing landscape of our skin's and body's health.

MEET YOUR SKIN

The skin is the most voluminous organ in the human body, comprising as much as 15 percent of the total adult body weight. A deeply sensitive and resilient organ, it protects against biological, chemical, mechanical, and ultraviolet threats. The skin serves as the medium between the outer world and our inner world.

Our skin is designed to:

- protect underlying tissues and organs from chemicals, microbes, and shock/impacts

- maintain body temperature by insulation (heating) and by sweat evaporation (cooling)

- synthesize and store vitamin D (converted to calcitriol for calcium regulation)

- protect the body from ultraviolet damage

- prevent excessive water loss

- store lipids (fats) in the dermis

- provide us with the ability to sense touch, pressure, pain, and temperature

- detox/excrete organic wastes, salt, and water

- serve as the first line of defense against pathogenic (disease-causing) microbes

- mediate the interrelationships between the immune, neurologic, and endocrine systems.

That's amazing! Now let's take a look at the structure of the skin. The skin consists of three major layers: the **epidermis**, the **dermis**, and the **hypodermis** (or subcutaneous tissue).

The epidermis, the top layer of the skin, is itself made up of four layers, with the exception of the palms of the hands and soles of the feet. They have a fifth layer known as the stratum lucidum, a thin, translucent superficial layer of extra protection due to the amount of tactile stimulation the hands and feet receive every day of our lives.

We will begin our journey with the stratum germinativum, the deepest, innermost layer of the epidermis.

Stratum Germinativum
(also called the basal cell layer)

The innermost layer of the epidermis, the part that connects with the dermis, is called the stratum germinativum, or the basal cell layer. The basal cells are responsible for actively producing new skin cells and then sending them on their journey, which can last up to 4 weeks, to the surface layer of the skin (the stratum corneum).

This layer includes melanocytes, cells that produce **melanin**, the pigment that colors our skin and hair as well as protects our skin from the sun's ultra-

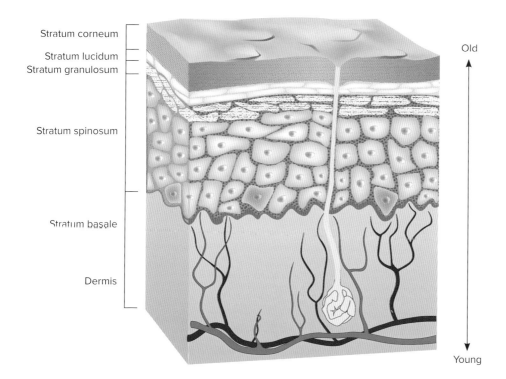

Stratum corneum

Stratum lucidum

Stratum granulosum

Stratum spinosum

Stratum basale

Dermis

Old

Young

STRUCTURE OF THE EPIDERMIS

violet radiation. It also includes **Merkel cells**, which produce the sensation of touch and are, not surprisingly, the most abundant in the hands and feet.

The potential impact of essential oils and carrier oils on this level of our skin includes support, enhancement of cellular rejuvenation (e.g., preventative to aging, wound healing), and protection from sun damage. This is also where the phototoxic aspects of essential oils such as bergamot and angelica root come into play.

Stratum Spinosum
(also called the squamous cell layer)

The stratum spinosum is the thickest layer of the epidermis and comprises of 5 to 10 cell layers. This layer has cells that contain special organelles called **lamellar bodies**. The lamellar bodies manufacture a wide variety of substances that deliver lipid precursors into the spaces between cells of the outer layer, the stratum corneum. As you will learn in a moment, lipids in the outer layer of the skin play a crucial role in the skin's barrier function.

Stratum Granulosum
(also called the Granular cell layer)

The stratum granulosum is the final layer of the epidermis that still contains living cells, although they are in transition. It is in this layer that living cells are dying, leaving behind keratin and keratohyalin, which form the stratum corneum. These cells also move up to form that fifth layer we mentioned, the stratum lucidum, which is found on the hands and feet.

Stratum Corneum
(also called the cornified or horny cell layer)

The outermost layer of our skin is called the stratum corneum. This layer is basically composed of non-living skin cells that are made up entirely of keratin protein. They are constantly being shed to make room for the new cells that work their way up from the lower layers of the epidermis. The stratum corneum is the layer of the epidermis that is directly exposed to the environment and is the layer to which we apply all kinds of body care products.

One of the major functions of our skin, specifically the stratum corneum, is to act as a physical and chemical barrier, preventing harmful substances and pathogens (microbes) from entering the skin as well as preventing excessive water loss. The metaphor of "brick-and-mortar" design is often used for the stratum corneum. But instead of mud and mortar holding the cells together, our skin uses lipids/fats, waxes, oils, proteins, and enzymes as the glue to hold the cells together and to nourish them. This mixture is called our **lipid matrix**, which is responsible for holding or binding moisture in between the "bricks," thus preventing water loss through the stratum corneum. Lipids also help lubricate the dry, dead cells, allowing our skin to be flexible.

The stratum corneum also contains the skin's natural moisturizing factor (NMF), a collection of water-soluble compounds responsible for keeping the skin moist and pliable by attracting water, either from the atmosphere or from products placed on the skin. The lipid matrix serves to prevent water loss from occurring in the NMF.

There is a saying in physiology that no part of the body should be dry. And by dry, we can mean two things: lack of water (dehydrated) and/or lack of oil (dry). Deficiency in either can affect this barrier function of the skin and increase water loss. The skin is constantly exposed to a variety of elements and influences including hot and cold temperatures, age, genetics, seasonal influences (e.g., heating during the winter months), and changing humidity levels. Excessive use of soap and other irritating chemicals can also break down the protective lipid layer and increase transepidermal water loss by altering the skin's natural water-holding capacity. The signs of a compromised skin barrier include dry, itchy, flaky, rough, and dull skin. The skin may also have fissures and cracks.

The topical application of vegetable oils, especially those rich in fatty acids and essential fatty acids, along with essential oils, can be of great benefit in restoring the skin barrier as well as in treating inflammatory disorders, eczema, dermatitis, and psoriasis; for wound healing; and for preventing wrinkles. The use of body scrubs and/or exfoliants can support the shedding of any dead cell build-up and promote the regeneration of cells in the stratum corneum and support its lipid matrix.

The Dermis

Sandwiched directly under the epidermis and above the subcutaneous layer is the dermis, the thickest layer of the skin. The dermis accounts for up to 90 percent of the total composition of the skin. The primary function of the **dermis** is to sustain and support the epidermis by providing physical and nutritional support. This section of the skin experiences a lot of activity. It's where our blood vessels, lymph glands, hair follicles, sebaceous and sweat glands, and all our sensory nerve cells live. Additionally, it's the location of connective fibers known as collagen and elastin, which give our skin flexibility and resiliency.

If essential oils, technically just some of their components, reach this layer of the skin, they may be picked up into the general blood and/or lymph circulation, whereby they will exert a subtle influence over our entire body.

The Hypodermis
(also called the subcutaneous layer)

Directly below the dermis is the hypodermis, also called the subcutaneous layer, which is composed mostly of fat cells. The main functions of this layer are stabilizing the skin, acting as a shock absorber and cushion for the vital internal organs, storing energy, and providing effective insulation.

Concerned about cellulite on the thighs? It's the hypodermis layer of the skin where we can find "cellulite," a common dimpling, puckering, and misshaping of the skin. Essential oils such as lemon and grapefruit, along with juniper berry, in a salt scrub could be incredibly beneficial for reducing the appearance of cellulite by promoting circulation and detoxification.

STRESS AND THE SKIN

Our skin is acutely sensitive to a variety of emotional states. Not only does it respond to our emotions and stress, but the appearance of our skin can itself cause or increase emotions or stress. Indeed, psychological stress has been shown to exacerbate acne, psoriasis, and other inflammatory skin conditions as well as reduce cellular rejuvenation and slow wound healing.

We may break out when we are stressed, or we appear dull and gray when we have not had enough sleep. "The skin is the mirror which reflects the state of the mind" has been a proverb since ancient times. The appearance and health of our skin can relate to our emotional state—along with diet and exercise, of course. And when any of these get thrown off balance, the skin is sure to reflect it.

Different skin conditions can also have a powerful impact on our social interactions, self-esteem, body image, and confidence. Psychological stress, therefore, can affect many aspects of the skin's function. Fortunately, essential oils are powerful allies in reducing the impact of stress and other emotional

imbalances that may arise from skin conditions or appearance. As you will learn in the next chapter on our sense of smell, aromatics and their ability to reduce stress have positive impacts on skin health.

Now that you understand how the skin is structured and its core functions, let's have a look at the ways in which essential oils are particularly suited for addressing a wide range of skin conditions.

Essential oils in body care products may be used to:

- enhance skin cell regeneration

- support the skin in fighting simple infections

- relieve itching due to dryness or insect bites

- reduce chronic or acute inflammation

- reduce the impact of stress on the skin

- enhance and support wound healing

- support the skin's barrier function and prevent water (moisture) loss, which is so vital for keeping the skin healthy

- reduce oiliness by supporting the regulation of sebum production

- minimize or slow aging of the skin

- protect from free-radical damage via their antioxidant activity

- relax and soothe emotions related to skin health and appearance.

In Part II we will be diving into more than 65 essential oils. The chart below is a summary of the core applications of essential oils for skin conditions, for supporting and enhancing the functions of the skin, and for the skin's overall health.

THERAPEUTIC BENEFITS AND ESSENTIAL OILS

ACTIVITY	ESSENTIAL OILS
Antimicrobial to support the skin in dealing with mild skin infections	Cistus, Geranium, Lavender, Lemon, Melissa, Niaouli, Palmarosa, Thyme ct. linalool
Reduce inflammation of eczema, psoriasis, insect bites, rosacea, mild burns, sunburn, etc.	Calendula CO_2, Cape Chamomile, German Chamomile, Roman Chamomile, Copaiba, Frankincense, Helichrysum, Lavender, Petitgrain, Sandalwood, Blue Tansy, Yarrow
Relieve itchiness	Cape Chamomile, German Chamomile, Lavender, Blue Tansy
Astringent-like for excess oil, acne	Himalayan Cedarwood, Cypress, Geranium, Neroli, Palmarosa, Patchouli, Rose
Cell regenerative as a preventative to aging and for skin rejuvenation	Calendula CO_2, Carrot Seed, Cistus, Frankincense, Helichrysum, Lavender, Myrrh, Neroli, Palmarosa, Patchouli, Rose, Yarrow
Emollient to soften and soothe skin	Carrier oils, herbal oils, creams, lotions
Wound healing including poorly or slowly healing wounds	Calendula CO_2, Carrot Seed, Cistus, Frankincense, Helichrysum, Lavender, Myrrh, Neroli, Palmarosa, Rose, Rosemary ct. verbenone, Yarrow
Nervine to reduce the impact of stress on the skin	Bergamot, Himalayan Cedarwood, Cape Chamomile, Roman Chamomile, German Chamomile, Frankincense, Lavender, Sweet Marjoram, Melissa, Neroli, Sweet Orange, Patchouli, Petitgrain, Rose, Sandalwood, Mandarin, Vetiver, Yarrow, Ylang Ylang

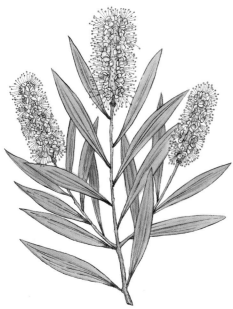

AROMATHERAPY FOR COMMON SKIN IMBALANCES

In this chart, we review common skin conditions, essential oils and other botanical ingredients that may be used for them, and the primary method of application. The carrier oils, herbal oils, hydrosols, and gels will be covered in more depth in chapter 6, and in chapter 7 you will learn how to make body care products.

COMMON SKIN CONDITIONS	ESSENTIAL OILS, CARRIER OILS, HERBAL OILS, AND HYDROSOLS
Inflamed Skin Conditions To calm and soothe inflammation	**Essential oils:** See essential oil chart above under "Reduces inflammation" **Carrier oils:** Jojoba, Neem, Pomegranate, Sea Buckthorn, Tamanu **Herbal oils:** Calendula **Hydrosols:** Lavender, German Chamomile, Helichrysum **Best body care products:** Cream, lotion, body or facial oil, gel, or body butter
Heat Rash Used to cool and calm inflammation	**Hydrosols:** German Chamomile, Lavender, Rose
Aging Skin Preventative for wrinkles and the damaging effects of free radicals, healing for sun damage	**Essential oils:** Calendula CO_2, Carrot Seed, Cistus, Frankincense, Helichrysum, Lavender, Myrrh, Neroli, Palmarosa, Patchouli, Rose, Yarrow **Carrier oils:** Avocado, Jojoba, Rosehip Seed, Tamanu **Herbal oils:** Calendula **Hydrosols:** German Chamomile, Helichrysum, Rose **Best body care products:** Cream, lotion, body or facial oil, or body butter
Itchy Skin **Common causes:** dry skin, bug bites / bed bugs, eczema (dermatitis), psoriasis, irritation, and allergies	**Essential oils:** Cape Chamomile, German Chamomile, Lavender, Blue Tansy **Carrier oils:** Baobab, Jojoba, Neem, Tamanu **Herbal oils:** Calendula **Hydrosols:** Calendula, German Chamomile, Lavender, Witch Hazel **Best body care products:** Spray hydrosol directly on affected area, apply aromatic gel, light cream or lotion, or body/facial oil
Dry Skin Remember that dry skin needs oil and/or water, both internally (via healthy diet and healthy fats) and externally	**Carrier oils:** Baobab, Borage Seed, Evening Primrose, Jojoba, Neem, Sesame, Pomegranate, Rosehip Seed, Tamanu **Herbal oils:** Calendula **Hydrosols:** Calendula, German Chamomile, Lavender **Best body care products:** unscented creams and lotions, body butters, and body or facial oils. With each of these products, spritz skin with a favorite hydrosol then apply the product

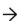

COMMON SKIN CONDITIONS	ESSENTIAL OILS, CARRIER OILS, HERBAL OILS, AND HYDROSOLS
Sunburn Hydrosols and Aloe Vera gel can provide relief from the initial sunburn	**Carrier oils:** Jojoba, Sunflower, Rosehip Seed, Tamanu **Herbal oils:** Calendula **Hydrosols:** Calendula, German Chamomile, Helichrysum, Lavender **Best body care products:** An aromatic gel. Spritzing the sunburn with hydrosols can be incredibly healing
Acne Used to reduce inflammation, address oil balance, address mild infection, if present, and soothe emotions	**Essential oils:** German Chamomile, Cape Chamomile, Blue Tansy, Lavender **Carrier oils:** Jojoba, Tamanu **Herbal oils:** Calendula **Hydrosols:** German Chamomile, Lavender, Helichrysum, Witch Hazel **Best body care products:** Facial or body cleanser, gel, hydrosols as toners
Cold Sores To support the body in healing	**Carrier oils:** Tamanu **Herbal oils:** St. John's Wort **Hydrosols:** Rose Geranium, Neroli, Witch Hazel **Best body care products:** Gel or carrier/herbal oil
First Aid To support wound cleaning and healing, reduce itchiness, and promote tissue healing	**Carrier oils:** Sea Buckthorn, Tamanu **Herbal oils:** Calendula, St. John's Wort **Hydrosols:** German Chamomile, Helichrysum, Lavender, Witch Hazel **Best body care products:** Aromatic gel

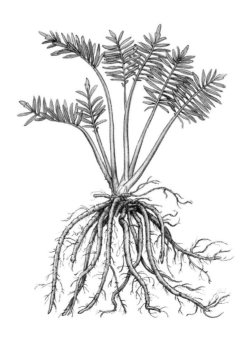

CHAPTER FOUR

OUR SENSE OF SMELL

PLANT-DERIVED AROMATICS can alter our perception, triggering memories and smell-related emotions and behaviors. They can also help regulate our appetite and physical responses, including our stress response. This wide range of potential effects is perhaps what makes aromatherapy one of the most inspiring holistic health modalities. Indeed, throughout history, humans have utilized plant aromatics for their physical and psychological benefits, from their euphoric and aphrodisiac properties to their stimulating and sedating properties.

Smell is a chemical sense, which means the receptors inside our nose respond to chemical stimuli. To arouse sensation, a substance must first be in a gaseous state before going into a mucous solution. The average healthy person can distinguish between ten and forty thousand odors (ad infinitum), many on a subliminal level. Smell relays messages from our outer world directly to the brain, influencing the physical body, mind, and emotions. That means our sense of smell is our first defense mechanism!

The olfactory system, our sense of smell, has direct access into the limbic system, also known as the emotional part of the brain. Olfactory nerves project directly into the amygdala without any mediation from the thalamus. It is only after the olfactory stimulus has reached the limbic system that it is sent to the frontal cortex for more associating, inhibiting, and other processing. This direct route is a result of the evolutionary role of the sense of smell. Olfactory nerve cells regenerate every 30 to 60 days, clearly underlining their importance. And although we do not use our sense of smell to quite the same extent that our ancestors did, it remains an important sense of sensation and healing.

The sense of smell is truly a wondrous sense, one that is often underutilized in our modern culture. However, the growing popularity of aromatherapy is bringing with it the awareness of this incredible sense.

According to the Sense of Smell Institute, as we enter the 21st century, fragrance (aromas) will be more than a glamorous fashion accessory or statement of personal style. They will be routinely used to:

- promote relaxation and reduce stress
- improve work performance
- elevate mood and reduce depression
- modify sleep and dreams
- enhance self-image
- retrieve memories
- enhance sexuality
- improve social relationships.[8]

And we are looking forward to it!

PATHWAY OF AN AROMA

Let's follow the scent of lavender as it wafts up into our nose. The nose is divided into two cavities by the nasal septum, and inside each nasal cavity are two parts: the olfactory part and the respiratory part.

The olfactory part of the nasal cavity is made up of the upper (superior) portion and a portion of the central section. The remaining tissue closer to the projection of the nose and a portion of the central section is the respiratory part. Sniffing increases the airflow through to the upper sinuses, thus increasing our perception of an aroma.

The respiratory part of the nasal cavity is lined with columnar and ciliated epithelium and is generously supplied with mucus-secreting goblet cells. Some of the aromatics or aromas inhaled will naturally follow the respiratory path into the lungs.

Let's continue our journey with our sense of smell. Once the aroma of lavender has been received by the olfactory epithelium, a nerve impulse is initiated into the olfactory bulb. Olfactory epithelium is a specialized epithelial tissue inside the nasal cavity that is involved in smell. The olfactory epithelium on each side of our nose is approximately the size of a small postage stamp. The olfactory epithelium in each nostril contains more than 3 to 5 million olfactory receptor cells (ORC). Olfactory epithelium regenerates every 30 to 60 days. This incredible ability of the olfactory tissue to reproduce nerve tissue illustrates its importance to human survival and the experience of living.

The olfactory bulb is continuous with the olfactory tract. The olfactory tract is a band of white matter that sends odor-related nerve impulses to the limbic system, beginning with the amygdala. Heavy innervation of the amygdala by primary olfactory structures provides a powerful mechanism for the rich experiences that can stem from olfactory sensation. The role of the amygdala in emotion, memory, and autonomic control directly ties olfaction to these primordial functions and adds complexity to the odor perceptual experience.[9]

The temporal and frontal lobes then interpret and perceive the odor. Thus, olfactory nerve projection encompasses the entire limbic region and associated pathways. Impulses that reach the limbic system activate smell-related emotions and behaviors.

As the aroma of lavender continues its journey via our sense of smell, it is capable of influencing our feelings, emotions, tension, and stress levels via its impact on the limbic system.

EXERCISE YOUR SENSE OF SMELL

The sense of smell, like muscles and the brain, needs exercise to become stronger. Often when someone thinks they don't have a good sense of smell, it is because they don't consciously use it. Also, some people don't like the smell of essential oils at first. Often this is because they have been brought up on synthetic odors and are used to the way synthetics smell. Usually, however, when they begin to exercise their sense of smell and become more familiar with the natural aromas of essential oils, they begin to experience the vast differences between synthetics and natural aromas.

To exercise your sense of smell, begin by simply observing different aromas/smells within your environment. Then move on to smelling plants when they are in bloom or natural, authentic essential oils. Take time to truly experience the nuances of an aroma. You could even keep a journal of all the different aromas you observe. Share your experiences with others.

Now, let's explore the limbic system. The limbic system consists of a number of structures located between the higher cerebral cortex and the lower brain including the amygdala, hypothalamus, and hippocampus, along with six other parts of the brain. We will focus our attention on these three.

The amygdala is the first part of the brain to register smell—in fact, it is only one synapse away! The amygdala is the integrative center for emotions, emotional behavior, and motivation. It is particularly involved with fear and anxiety, and it plays a central role in aggression. It also plays a role in male sexual motivation. Our sense of smell has direct access to the amygdala and thus can potentially interrupt the stress response at this level, decreasing the potentially negative impact of stress or anxiety. It makes sense that aromatics such as essential oils can modify or influence our emotions and behavior!

The hypothalamus lies below the thalamus and above the pituitary gland in the heart of the brain. The hypothalamus is partly under the control of the prefrontal lobes and is intimately connected with the limbic system. The main function of the hypothalamus is homeostasis or maintaining the body's status quo. The three major systems controlled by the hypothalamus for maintenance of homeostasis (and allostasis) are the autonomic nervous system, the neuroendocrine system, and the limbic system.

The hippocampus is a curved band of gray matter that is involved with learning and memory. It is vital for short-term memory as well as for the consolidation of that memory into a long-term form. It has been shown that the hippocampus shrinks in size when an individual is under stress. Ahhh! That's another reason aromatics are so powerful. They can reduce the impact of stress while improving memory formation and longevity.

In general terms, the limbic system makes rapid parallel decisions integrating the necessary parts of the central nervous system and the body required for any decision. Externally the limbic system supports eating, copulating, and fighting. Internally the limbic system directs body posture for food, sexual activity, or sleep, and it controls internal viscera and hormones. It has specific areas that govern mood and feeling states. Overall the limbic system is a complex internal sensory system orchestrating the various parts of the body. Returning to our example of lavender, we can see that simply by smelling an essential oil (its aroma), it can reduce the impact of stress, soothe and relax the body, and support resiliency against stress. Indeed, our sense of smell and aromatics are powerful inputs to it, capable of influencing our emotions and motivating us to move.

WHAT DETERMINES OUR GENERAL REACTION TO A PARTICULAR AROMA?

Aromas do not by definition have a positive or negative influence, nor does a specific aroma elicit a specific mood. Smell-evoked emotions and behavior evolve out of experiences that occur in the presence of those aromas. For an aroma to have meaning, an individual must develop a relationship with it based upon associations and actual experiences. Some factors that determine our general reaction to an aroma or smell are:

- previous experience of that aroma or one of a similar aroma

- our current emotional state when exposed to the odor/aroma

- whether the aroma is perceived as pleasant or unpleasant

- any auto-suggested relations (e.g., this oil is known to be relaxing or anxiety relieving)

- most importantly, the environment in which the aroma is introduced.

THE HEALING POWERS OF AROMA

Now that we've explored the power of our sense of smell, let's look at what potential benefits essential oils have when we're utilizing it. Aromatics (e.g., essential oils, CO_2s, and absolutes) can:

- reduce or alleviate stress and anxiety

- relieve pain by altering pain perception in the brain

- induce sleep or relaxation

- increase alertness and overall performance

- be used for weight control or loss

- help alleviate nausea

- affect and improve mood and increase overall emotional well-being

- be a useful stress management tool due to impact on the autonomic nervous system

- ease physical ailments, particularly stress-related disorders

- help shape our impressions of self and others.

In the next chapter, we will be covering individual essential oils and sharing their potential applications for a range of emotions. In chapter 8, we will review the various methods of application that are used specifically for our sense of smell, although all body care products containing essential oils are capable of affecting our emotional well-being through the sense of smell as well. But first, here are a few recipes that reveal the potential of essential oils to affect our emotional and physical well-being.

AROMATIC MEMORIES

Aromas can stir up lost memories and emotions. In fact, memories attached to a particular aroma or smell are considered to be some of the longest lasting forms of memory. For example, the smell of apple pie baking may remind you of being at home with your family, and you may feel comforted by this aroma. On the other hand, an antiseptic-type aroma may remind you of being in a hospital when you or someone in your family was sick. Memories can have both positive and negative connotations. Take a moment to reflect on memories and emotions you have that are related to a specific aroma or smell.

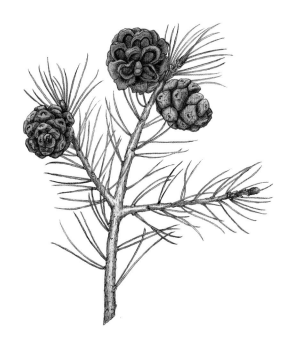

→ Sleepy Time Diffuser Blend for Insomnia

AUTHOR: Elisabeth Vlasic

Diffusing calming essential oils at night is a restorative way to prepare one's body for sleep. It will surely become a comforting part of your regular nighttime ritual! This blend is made up of the mother of all essential oils, lavender, as well as both Roman and German chamomile. This is a classically gentle, yet effective remedy heralded for its soothing and relaxing benefits. It is also safe for children.

Prep Time: 15 minutes
Yield: Approximately 1 teaspoon (5 ml)
Safety: No known concerns

INGREDIENTS
- 56 drops Lavender (*Lavandula angustifolia*) essential oil
- 7 drops Roman Chamomile (*Chamaemelum nobile)* essential oil
- 7 drops German Chamomile (*Matricaria chamomilla* syn. *Matricaria recutita*) essential oil

WHAT YOU NEED
- A small glass or stainless-steel bowl
- Glass, stainless-steel, or wooden stirrer
- 5 ml empty, dark-colored bottle with orifice reducer
- Plastic or glass pipette
- Label

PROCEDURE
1. Place lavender, Roman chamomile, and German chamomile essential oils in a bowl.

2. Gently stir, ensuring the essential oils mix together well.

3. Using a pipette, fill the bottle with the blend.

4. Add orifice reducer, cap tightly, and label.

How to use the Sleepy Time Diffuser Blend:
Following diffuser manufacturer instructions, add Sleepy Time Diffuser Blend to a diffuser and turn on 5 minutes before entering the room to sleep. If you do not have a diffuser, you can place a few drops of the blend on your pillow and/or bedsheets, on a tissue to hold to your nose to breathe in, or on the inside corner of your clothing.

ALTERNATE ESSENTIAL OILS: (can be used at same number of drops as recipe): Bergamot (*Citrus bergamia*), Clary Sage (*Salvia sclarea*), and Sweet Marjoram (*Origanum majorana*).

NOTE: Drop size varies. It will generally take 77 to 120 drops to fill a 5 ml bottle. This recipe is an estimate for filling your 5 ml bottle. You can always add or decrease the individual drops as you deem fit for your personal use.

✈ Tension Release Spritzer

AUTHOR: Amy Anthony

Hypertension may be caused by many things, including stress. Working with essential oils known to calm and relax the nerves and dilate blood vessels may be helpful for anyone living with tension impacting the cardiovascular system. Ylang ylang and khella are classic hypotensive and opening oils, while valerian and vetiver provide grounding and nerve calming properties. These are all supported by coriander's propensity to dispel nervous exhaustion.

Prep Time: 5 minutes
Yield: Approximately 2 ounces (60 ml)
Safety: Khella may be photosensitizing for some people. Take care with sun exposure if using this recipe, though the minimal amount of khella that will come out of the spritzer in each spray may not be of much concern.

INGREDIENTS
- 16 drops Coriander (*Coriandrum sativum*) essential oil
- 10 drops Ylang Ylang Complete (*Cananga odorata*) essential oil
- 2 drops Khella (*Ammi visnaga*) essential oil
- 1 drop Valerian (*Valeriana officinalis*) essential oil
- 1 drop Vetiver (*Chrysopogon (Vetiveria) zizanioides*) essential oil
- 2 ounces (60 ml) distilled water or Lavender hydrosol

WHAT YOU NEED
- Measuring cup or beaker
- 2 ounces (60 ml) glass or PET (polyethylene terephthalate) bottle with spray top
- Label

PROCEDURE
1. Pour the distilled water into a 2-ounce (60 ml) bottle.

2. Add essential oils, affix the spray top, and label.

How to use the Tension Release Aromatic Spritzer: Shake the bottle before using to disperse the essential oils into the distilled water. There are many options for using the spritzer. Use as needed, within 3 months.

- Spray the air in front of you 2 to 3 times and walk through the mist, keeping your eyes closed.

- Spray your clothing 2 to 3 times and enjoy the effect of the aroma.

- Spray 2 to 3 times directly onto your pillow before going to sleep.

NOTE: This is blended at a 2.5 percent dilution (30 drops of essential oil in a 2-ounce [60 ml] product), which is indicated for general holistic aromatherapy.

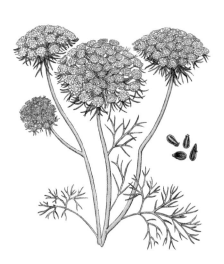

⇢ Self-Love Botanical Perfume

AUTHOR: Elisabeth Vlasic

Oh, the joy of becoming a parent. While some women have immediate ease in this area, obtaining a pregnancy is not as easy for others. It can be a challenging time in a woman's life, with feelings of uncertainty on the journey to a hopefully positive test result. We have all heard urban myths of women trying for many years to get pregnant, giving up, adopting a puppy or kitten instead, and miraculously falling pregnant. Yes, falling pregnant and stress go hand in hand. Once you let that stress go, miracles can happen. One of the characteristics of essential oils is that they can alleviate stress in the body and mind, and with stress playing a part in hormonal balance, our Self-Love Botanical Perfume is an intentional talisman to soothe the spirit.

This decadent, nurturing botanical perfume offers support, reminding the wearer to love herself and bringing inner calm and peace. It's a heavenly combination of rose, neroli, ravintsara ct. cineole (ho leaf), frankincense, and jasmine.

Yield: Approximately 1 teaspoon (5 ml)
Prep Time: 25 minutes
Safety: No concerns.

INGREDIENTS
- 1 drop Rose (*Rosa × damascene*) essential oil
- 2 drops Neroli (*Citrus aurantium var. amara*) essential oil
- 1 drop Ravintsara ct. cineole (*Cinnamomum camphora*) essential oil
- 4 drops Frankincense (*Boswellia sacra*) essential oil
- 1 drop Jasmine (*Jasminum grandiflorum*) essential oil
- Just under 2 teaspoons (10 ml) Jojoba (*Simmondsia chinensis*)

WHAT YOU NEED
- A small glass beaker or stainless-steel bowl
- Glass, stainless steel, or wooden stirrer/spoon
- Pipette
- 10 ml roller bottle
- Label

PROCEDURE
1. Place rose, neroli, ravintsara ct. cineole, frankincense, and jasmine essential oils into the glass beaker.

2. Gently stir, ensuring the essential oils mix together well.

3. Add jojoba to the beaker and stir well, incorporating the essential oils thoroughly.

4. Either carefully pour or pipette the oil mixture into the bottle.

5. Add the insert and ball, cap tightly, and label.

How to use Self-Love Botanical Perfume:
Anoint the preferred perfume points on the body throughout the day, taking a moment to think positively about one's goal of falling pregnant—inner wrists, behind ear lobes, and at the base of the throat.

ALTERNATE ESSENTIAL OILS: Clary Sage (*Salvia sclarea*), Melissa (*Melissa officinalis*), and Ylang Ylang (*Cananga odorata*).

NOTE: The essential oil blend in this recipe is created on a 5 percent dilution, as it is for a perfume.

PART III

The Essential Apothecary

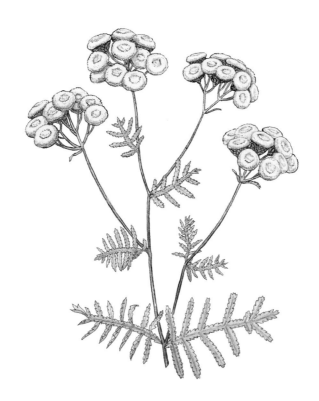

CHAPTER FIVE

THE ESSENTIAL OILS

ESSENTIAL OILS are at the very heart of aromatherapy. These plant-derived aromatics not only support our health and well-being, but they also help us to take care of ourselves during times of ill health and emotional stress.

In this chapter we will be covering more than 60 essential oils. That's a lot of essential oils! It takes time to get to know each individual one. Cultivating a personal relationship with each essential oil provides you with the confidence and empowerment you need to use them for a wide range of health conditions and imbalances.

Each essential oil mini-monograph contains the following information:

COMMON NAME (LATIN NAME, BOTANICAL FAMILY)
Angelica Root (*Angelica archangelica*, Apiaceae)

The common name is the most widely accepted name for a given plant species within a given culture or region. The binomial Latin name, also called the scientific name, is the internationally recognized identity of a specific plant, distinguishing it from all others. Why is this important? Because, for example, there are more than 700 species in the *Eucalyptus* genus, of which eight are commonly found within the aromatherapy industry. These are *Eucalyptus globulus, Eucalyptus dives, Eucalyptus (Corymbia) citriodora, Eucalyptus staigeriana,*

Eucalyptus smithii, Eucalyptus camaldulensis, Eucalyptus polybractea, and *Eucalyptus radiata.* Although they share some common therapeutic benefits, each species has its own individual chemistry and "personality" and therefore unique therapeutic applications.

Knowing the common and Latin name of the plants in each essential oil you purchase is, therefore, important.

PART OF PLANT: The initial paragraph in each mini-monograph contains the part of plant used in producing the essential oil.

A good example of why the part of the plant is important is the bitter orange tree, *Citrus aurantium* var. *amara.* Three different essential oils are produced from three different parts of this tree: Petitgrain from the leaves, Neroli from orange blossoms, and Bitter Orange from the zest of the fruit. When a plant produces essential oils in more than one of its parts, differences in aroma and chemical composition occur.

SOURCE COUNTRIES: These are the countries where the essential oil is typically distilled and sourced.

CORE COMPONENTS: This section provides the core components of the essential oil.

NOTE: CHEMOTYPES

Many factors influence the chemical composition of essential oils, including growing conditions of the plant such as light, soil, temperature, moisture, climate, and altitude, as well its geographic area (country of origin). The term *chemotype* is used to describe an essential oil that has been extracted from one botanical species yet varies considerably from the norm in chemical composition.

Let's take a closer look at what this means. The two most commonly available essential oils that have a number of different chemotypes are rosemary and thyme. Some essential oils are available only with one chemotype commonly available—for example Niaouli ct. cineole. A chemotype will be noted with the abbreviation "ct.", as in Rosemary ct. verbenone or Thyme ct. linalool. When purchasing essential oils, be sure you know which chemotype you are receiving.

SAFETY: This section provides safety information relevant to the application of essential oils to the skin, via inhalation, or via diffusion. This section does not contain information relevant to the internal use of essential oils.

CONSERVATION: The conservation status informs us to what degree a plant is likely to become extinct in the wild. The medicinal use of plants is partially responsible for the depletion and even extinction of some wild plants. Information on conservation status is taken from the International Union for Conservation of Nature's (IUCN) Red List of Threatened Species, which defines extinction risk using criteria such as areas of occupancy, population numbers, reproductive rate and success, current and projected threats to the species and its habitat, and so on.

Conservation status ranges from Least Concern, which means the plant is not threatened, all the way to Extinct, meaning it has, tragically, disappeared completely. In between these extremes are Near Threatened, Vulnerable, Endangered, Critically Endangered, and Extinct in the Wild.

Those essential oils which are noted as "Not defined" are most likely on the least concerned list but be sure to check the IUCN website for the most up-to-date information.

BLENDING WITH THE ESSENTIAL OIL

This section includes information of value when blending with the specific essential oil. This information includes:

- **Aroma:** core words used to describe the aroma of the essential oil

- **System affinities:** the core systems of the body that the essential oil has an affinity with

- **Blends well with:** a list of essential oils that blend well with the essential oil being covered. This list is a starting point and is not meant to be exhaustive.

- **Potential substitutions:** some ideas on potential substitutions for the essential oil. At times, it may require two essential oils to achieve the same therapeutic activity. We recommend equal drops between the essential oils given. These combinations have been included.

THERAPEUTIC APPLICATIONS

This section focuses on the system affinity of the essential oil, along with its psyche/emotional benefits.

- **Indications:** This section highlights indications broken down into different systems of the body. The indications are not meant to be exhaustive. In this section we also include other systems of

ABOUT SYSTEM AFFINITIES

If you have ever read an aromatherapy book or taken a class, you may have encountered so many therapeutic applications for each essential oil that it's challenging to figure out which oil to select for which imbalance or condition, and if it even matters. Well, it can. We, on the other hand, believe that each essential oil has very specific affinities to systems of the body, or at times to one specific system of the body. And although each essential oil we cover is capable of affecting a variety of systems, we've chosen to focus on what that essential oil is the best at. We've taken into account its chemistry, history, and herbal use, as well as our experience and research to narrow this down. We've also taken into consideration its nature as a plant and what it has historically had an affinity to. Please remember though, this is not meant to exclude all the other things an individual essential oil is capable of. It is meant as a starting point to get to know the heart of that essential oil and then you can move freely around and beyond.

PSYCHE/EMOTIONS

Regardless of the system of the body you are addressing, all aromatherapy products applied to the skin, for the skin's health or for another body system, or used via inhalation or diffusion, will naturally affect the mind and emotions. We did not include this in the Specific Affinity section because all essential oils, by their very nature, can influence how we feel or alter the landscape of our stress response. There are, however, some essential oils—such as tea tree or winter savory—that are never used for their olfactory (sense of smell) potential. Even though they will have some kind of impact, they are just simply not used that way. They are used more for their broad spectrum antimicrobial activity, which is not system-specific.

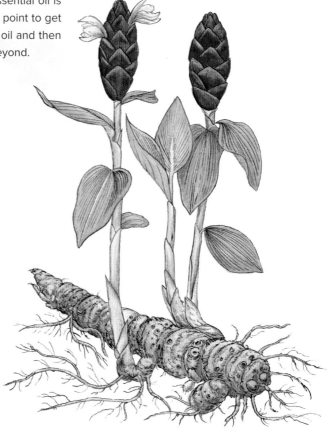

OXIDIZING OILS

Throughout the essential oil mini-monographs, you will come across safety messages regarding when certain essential oils oxidize. What happens when an essential oil oxidizes? And how do you know when it does? There are certain components (e.g., some monoterpenes or the monoterpene alcohol, linalool) that, over time and as they are exposed to air, become oxidized.

Unfortunately, it can be challenging to know when an essential oil oxidizes. Often skin irritation can be the first sign. Other potential signs include a change in the aroma. Just think about how we know when food or carrier oils have gone off. They begin to smell differently—sometimes downright horrible. With essential oils, the aroma may begin to change as it oxidizes, and it may begin to thicken or become more viscous.

For essential oils that have this concern, the dermal safety note will state, "Oxidized citrus essential oils, such as bergamot, should not be used in body care products for application to the skin. The essential oil can, however, be used for cleaning products."

Once again, the shelf lives of essential oils from chapter 2 are:

* *For monoterpene-rich essential oils*, 1 to 2 years, e.g., citrus oils, conifers (Scots Pine, Hemlock Spruce), Frankincense, Lemongrass, and Neroli

* *For all other essential oils:* 2 to 3 years

* *For viscous essential oils*, e.g., Vetiver, Patchouli, and Sandalwood: 4 to 8+ years

the body that, although they may not be core system affinities, are still systems we would think about for that specific essential oil, mostly as a support essential oil.

- **Method of application:** These are the recommended methods of application for the system. Please note that the term *personal inhaler* includes an alternative to plastic—smelling salts.

- **Pairs well with:** This list categorizes the above "Blends well with" essential oils into specific systems of the body they have an affinity within their support of the primary essential oil.

Now, on to the exciting part: getting to know the essential oils! We are about to dive into specific essential oils. Some you may have, some you may be ordering, and some you may hope one day to purchase (e.g., rose essential oil; it's expensive!). We recommend getting any that you do own out while reading about them.

Here's our approach to getting to know an essential oil through our nose, our sense of smell. Begin with the awareness that essential oils are very powerful, and each of us has a different level of sensitivity when it comes to aromas. Hold the open bottle approximately 4 to 5 inches (10 to 13 cm) away from your nose, then move it closer as needed to get the full aroma. As you hold the bottle of essential oil below your nose, gently move it back and forth between your left and right nostrils. This way you will receive the full spectrum of aroma the oil has to give. The aroma should continue to expand as you continue to smell. Pay attention to its several layers. This process only takes a minute or two, but it is the beginning of developing your olfactory palate, so to speak. Now, onwards to the essential oils.

BLACK PEPPER

Distilled using dried black peppercorns, **Black Pepper** (*Piper nigrum*, Piperaceae) essential oil shines in its ability to support healthy circulation and digestion. Warm and spicy, black pepper essential oil also has pain relieving activity, making it a great addition to muscular aches and pains remedies. The aroma of black pepper seems to be all about the will, strength, and empowerment.

SOURCE COUNTRIES: India, Indonesia, Brazil, Malaysia, Thailand, Sri Lanka, and Madagascar

CORE COMPONENTS: β-caryophyllene, limonene, β-pinene, α-pinene

DERMAL CAUTION: Potential skin sensitizer if the oil is oxidized. The shelf life is 1 to 2 years. Avoid older oils and store correctly.

CONSERVATION: Not yet assessed

BLENDING WITH BLACK PEPPER

AROMA: Pungent, peppery, spicy, warming

SYSTEM AFFINITIES: Circulatory, digestive, musculoskeletal

BLENDS WELL WITH: Carrot Seed, Clove, Sweet Fennel, Ginger, Grapefruit, Laurel, Lemon, Mandarin, Neroli, Niaouli, Rose, Rosemary ct. cineole or Rosemary ct. camphor, Sweet Marjoram

THERAPEUTIC APPLICATIONS

INDICATIONS	METHOD OF APPLICATION	PAIRS WELL WITH
Circulatory system: Poor circulation, Raynaud's syndrome, sensitivity to cold	Salt scrub, unscented cream or lotion, body oil	Carrot Seed, Ginger, Grapefruit, Lemon, Rose
Digestive system: Indigestion, excess gas, sluggish digestion, lack of appetite	Personal inhaler, salt inhaler, abdominal oil, diffuser	Sweet Fennel, Ginger, Grapefruit, Lemon
Musculoskeletal system: Muscular aches and pains, rheumatism, muscle stiffness, arthritic pain	Body oil, gel, aromatic bath, salve	Clary Sage, Laurel, Lavender, Lemon, Sweet Marjoram, Rosemary ct. camphor or Rosemary ct. cineole
Psyche/emotions: Mental fatigue, emotional coldness, apathy, low endurance, nervousness, weakness of will, loss of motivation, emotional exhaustion, indecisiveness	Personal inhaler, aromatic bath, diffuser	Grapefruit, Juniper Berry, Lemon, Peppermint, Rose, Rosemary ct. cineole

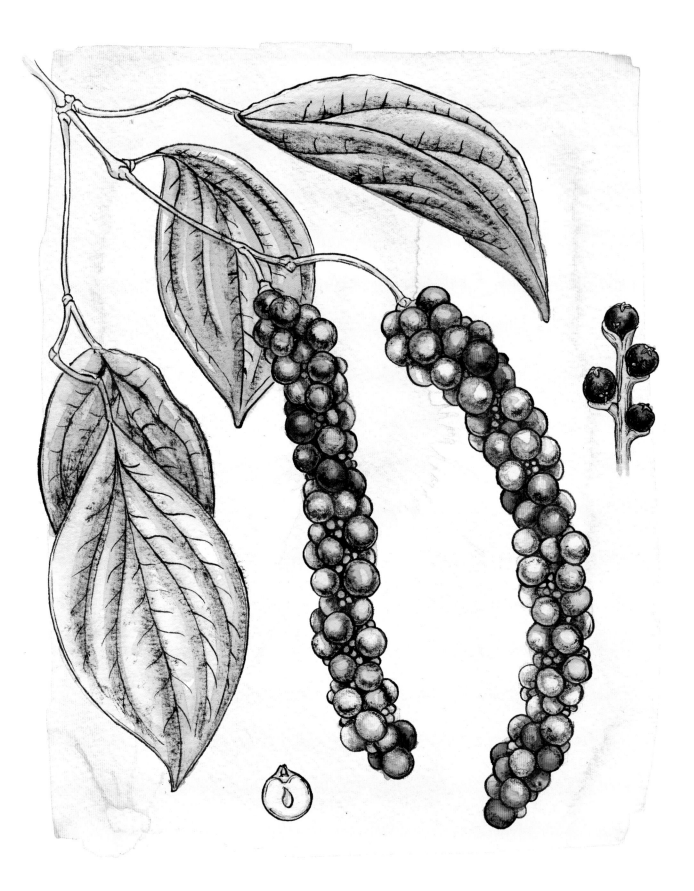

CYPRESS

Cypress (*Cupressus sempervirens*, Cupressaceae) essential oil is extracted from the leaves, twigs, and cones of the cypress tree via steam distillation. Prized for its astringent-like qualities, cypress shines in remedies for varicose veins or skin conditions caused by excess oil (sebum). With its affinity to the respiratory system, cypress can reduce spasmodic coughs and support the body in fighting respiratory infections.

SOURCE COUNTRIES: France and Italy

CORE COMPONENTS: α-pinene, α-cedrol, delta-3-carene, and other monoterpenes

DERMAL CAUTION: Due to the monoterpene content, it is important to store the essential oil properly (in a dark container in the refrigerator or in a cold room away from sunlight and heat). Oxidized essential oils should not be used in body care products or in formulations designed for dermal application. This essential oil can, however, be used for cleaning products.

CONSERVATION: Least concern

BLENDING WITH CYPRESS

AROMA: Piney, woody, refreshing

SYSTEM AFFINITIES: Respiratory, circulatory, skin

BLENDS WELL WITH: Bergamot, Black Pepper, Cedarwood, Clary Sage, Geranium, Helichrysum, Juniper Berry, Lavender, Lemon, Sweet Marjoram, Niaouli, Rose, Rosemary, Saro, Black Spruce

POTENTIAL SUBSTITUTIONS: Geranium, Lemon, Rose

THERAPEUTIC APPLICATIONS

INDICATIONS	METHOD OF APPLICATION	PAIRS WELL WITH
Circulatory system: Varicose veins, cellulite	Salt scrub (cellulite), gel (varicose veins)	Grapefruit, Helichrysum (varicose veins in gel), Juniper Berry, Lemon
Respiratory system: Coughs, particularly spasmodic dry coughs, bronchitis, asthma, flu, sore throat	Chest salve, undiluted on neck/throat area (sore throats)	Black Pepper, Cedarwood, Juniper Berry, Lavender, Sweet Marjoram, Niaouli, Rosemary ct. cineole, Saro
Skin: Oily, sweaty skin and feet, broken capillaries, rosacea, bruises, cellulite, excessive sweating	Facial or body cleanser, gel, unscented cream or lotion	Cedarwood, Geranium, Lemon, Rose
Psyche/emotions: Anxiety, excessive talking, excessive thinking. Deepens yet contracts the breath. Calming, helpful during times of transition and bereavement	Personal inhaler, diffuser, nebulizing diffuser, aromatic baths	Bergamot, Black Pepper, Cedarwood, Clary Sage, Geranium, Lavender, Sweet Marjoram, Rose, Black Spruce

JUNIPER BERRY

Juniper Berry (*Juniperus communis*, Cupressaceae) essential oil is steam distilled using juniper berries and is much prized for its awakening and inspiring aroma.

SOURCE COUNTRIES: Countries of the Balkans, France, and Italy

CORE COMPONENTS: α-pinene, β-myrcene, germacrene D

SAFETY: Due to the monoterpene content, it is important that the essential oil be stored properly (in a dark container in the refrigerator or in a cold room away from sunlight and heat). Oxidized essential oils should not be used in body care products or formulations designed for dermal application. The essential oil can, however, be used for cleaning products.

CONSERVATION: Not yet assessed

BLENDING WITH JUNIPER BERRY

AROMA: Fresh, piney, fruity

SYSTEM AFFINITIES: Circulatory, musculoskeletal

BLENDS WELL WITH: Carrot Seed, Clary Sage, Cypress, Himalayan Cedarwood, Blue Gum Eucalyptus, Ginger, Grapefruit, Lavender, Lemon, Lemongrass, Palmarosa, Sweet Marjoram, Rosemary ct. cineole

POTENTIAL SUBSTITUTIONS: Grapefruit, Lemon, Blue Gum Eucalyptus

THERAPEUTIC APPLICATIONS

INDICATIONS	METHOD OF APPLICATION	PAIRS WELL WITH
Circulatory system: Poor circulation	Salt scrub	Blue Gum Eucalyptus, Ginger, Grapefruit, Lemon, Lemongrass, Rosemary ct. cineole
Musculoskeletal system: Muscular aches and pains, rheumatism, cellulite, joint pain and stiffness, strains and sprains, carpal tunnel syndrome, sciatica, spasms, edema	Body oil, salve, aromatic baths (with sea salts or magnesium salts)	Clary Sage, Cypress, Himalayan Cedarwood, Ginger, Grapefruit, Lavender, Lemon, Lemongrass, Sweet Marjoram, Rosemary ct. cineole
Psyche/emotions: Fluctuating energy levels, worry, cold, fear, trembling, feelings of being blocked, lack of motivation	Personal inhaler, foot baths	Clary Sage, Cypress, Himalayan Cedarwood, Ginger, Grapefruit, Lavender, Lemon, Sweet Marjoram, Rosemary ct. cineole

ROSE

The aromatics of **Rose** (*Rosa x damascene*, Rosaceae) petals can be extracted via hydro-distillation (essential oil), carbon dioxide hypercritical extraction (CO_2 extract), or solvent extraction (absolute). Considered the queen of essential oils, it is often used with emotional imbalances related to menstruation, perimenopause, and menopause. Rose also shines in facial care products. Rose can lift one out of mild depression or help process grief.

SOURCE COUNTRIES: Bulgaria, Morocco, Turkey, and India

CORE COMPONENTS: Essential oil: citronellol, nerol, geraniol; Absolute: phenylethanol, citronellol, geraniol, nerol

SAFETY: No known contraindications or cautions

CONSERVATION: Not defined

BLENDING WITH ROSE

AROMA: Floral, rich, warm, feminine

SYSTEM AFFINITIES: Female and male reproductive, skin, psyche/emotion

BLENDS WELL WITH: Angelica Root, Bergamot Mint, Black Pepper, Cardamom, Coriander Seed, Celery Seed, Cypress, Sweet Fennel, Grapefruit, Ginger, Himalayan Cedarwood, Katafray, Lemon, Myrrh, Mandarin, Sweet Marjoram, Neroli, Sweet Orange, Palmarosa, Pink Pepper, Plai, Thyme ct. linalool, Valerian, Ylang Ylang

POTENTIAL SUBSTITUTIONS: Ylang Ylang, Neroli, Jasmine, Rose Geranium

THERAPEUTIC APPLICATIONS

INDICATIONS	METHOD OF APPLICATION	PAIRS WELL WITH
Circulatory system: Varicose veins, broken capillaries	Gel, body oil, cream	Cypress, Lemon, Myrrh, Neroli, Palmarosa
Reproductive system: Irregular/painful menstruation, impotence, sterility, frigidity, reduced/low libido, PMS, amenorrhea, menopause, mild postnatal depression	Personal inhaler, aromatic baths, abdominal oil, body oil	Sweet Fennel, Grapefruit, Mandarin, Sweet Marjoram, Neroli, Sweet Orange, Plai, Valerian, Ylang Ylang
Skin: Broken capillaries, oily skin, mature and sensitive skin, aging skin, wounds, skin blotches, rosacea.	Cream, facial oil, gel	Cypress, Lemon, Myrrh, Neroli, Palmarosa
Psyche/emotions: Depression, insomnia, shock, anxiety, grief, mood swings, frigidity, lack of libido, heartbreak, anger, frustration, jealousy, resentment, difficulty loving or trusting, lack of creativity	Personal inhaler, roll-on, aromatic bath	Angelica Root, Bergamot Mint, Cardamom, Coriander Seed, Celery Seed, Grapefruit, Myrrh, Mandarin, Neroli, Sweet Orange, Pink Pepper, Valerian, Ylang Ylang

VALERIAN

Valerian (*Valeriana officinalis*, Caprifoliaceae) essential oil is steam distilled using the rhizomes (like roots) of valerian. It offers a unique aroma that can lure one to sleep or simply calm and soothe one's spirits after a long day's work.

SOURCE COUNTRY: Nepal

CORE COMPONENTS: Bornyl acetate, myrtenyl acetate, valerianol, valeranone, camphene, α-pinene, allo-aromadendrene

SAFETY: No known cautions or contraindications

CONSERVATION: Not yet assessed

BLENDING WITH VALERIAN

AROMA: Sweet-woody, earthy, sensual

SYSTEM AFFINITIES: Digestive

BLENDS WELL WITH: Angelica Root, Roman Chamomile, Copaiba, Coriander Seed, Cypress, Cistus, Grapefruit, Lavender, Lemon, Mandarin, Sweet Marjoram, Neroli, Pinyon Pine, Vetiver, Ylang Ylang

POTENTIAL SUBSTITUTIONS: Roman Chamomile, Vetiver, Ginger

THERAPEUTIC APPLICATIONS

INDICATIONS	METHOD OF APPLICATION	PAIRS WELL WITH:
Digestive system: Nervous indigestion or other digestive issues that arise from stress	Personal inhaler, roll-on	Roman Chamomile, Coriander Seed, Grapefruit, Lavender, Lemon
Psyche/emotions: Insomnia, agitation, nervous fatigue, irritability, fatigue	Personal inhaler, roll-on, aromatic bath	Angelica Root, Roman Chamomile, Copaiba, Coriander Seed, Cypress, Cistus, Grapefruit, Lavender, Lemon, Mandarin, Sweet Marjoram, Neroli, Pinyon Pine, Vetiver, Ylang Ylang

ANGELICA ROOT

Angelica Root (*Angelica archangelica*, Apiaceae) essential oil is steam distilled using the dried roots of the angelica plant. As a root essential oil, angelica is exceptional for its ability to ground and center one when one is feeling overwhelmed or a bit anxious. Angelica root is the essential oil for supporting and building resilience by keeping one rooted in one's life.

SOURCE COUNTRIES: China, France, India, and Germany

CORE COMPONENTS: Rich in monoterpenes (α-pinene, α-phellandrene, β-phellandrene, myrcene, sabinene, d-limonene). Important trace component: angelicin, which is responsible for the phototoxicity of angelica root.

SAFETY: Photosensitizer. The recommended dilution to avoid damage from the sun is approximately one drop of essential oil per 1⅓ teaspoons (6.6 ml) of vegetable or other carrier oil, cream, or gel. We recommend avoiding application to the skin if going into the sun.

CONSERVATION: Least concern

BLENDING WITH ANGELICA ROOT

AROMA: Sweet, rich herbaceous, earthy, musky, woody

SYSTEM AFFINITIES: Digestive

BLENDS WELL WITH: Bergamot, Black Pepper, Copaiba, Coriander Seed, Fingerroot, Geranium, Jasmine Absolute, Katafray, Lavender, Lemon, Mandarin, Neroli, Sweet Orange, Patchouli, Petitgrain, Rose, Vetiver, Ylang Ylang

POTENTIAL SUBSTITUTIONS: Lavender + Lemon + Ginger, Sweet Fennel + Grapefruit, Celery Seed + Katafray

THERAPEUTIC APPLICATIONS

INDICATIONS	METHOD OF APPLICATION	PAIRS WELL WITH
Digestive system: Indigestion, excess gas, sluggish digestion, lack of appetite, stress-related digestive upsets	Personal inhaler, abdominal oil*	Bergamot, Black Pepper, Coriander Seed, Fingerroot, Ginger, Grapefruit, Lavender, Lemon
Psyche/emotions: Nervous tension or upset, irritability, anxiety, insomnia, nervousness, sleep disturbances, emotional ups and downs, feelings of being overwhelmed	Roll-on*, body oil*, personal inhaler, aromatic baths* *Refer to safety information above.	Bergamot, Coriander Seed, Geranium, Jasmine Absolute, Katafray, Lavender, Lemon, Mandarin, Neroli, Sweet Orange, Patchouli, Petitgrain, Rose, Vetiver, Ylang Ylang

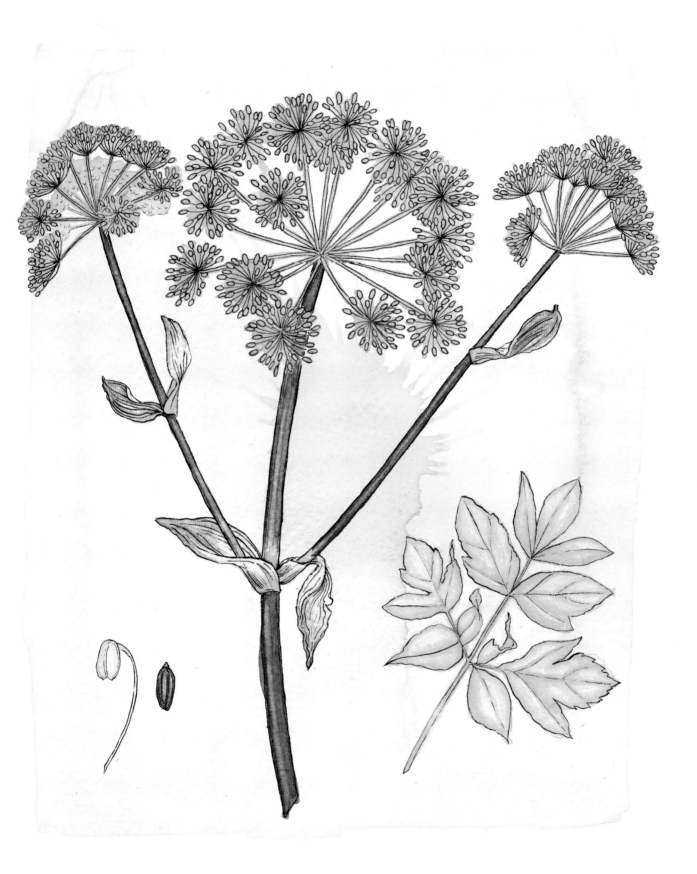

ANISE

Indigenous to the Mediterranean region, **Anise** (*Pimpinella anisum*, Apiaceae) essential oil is steam distilled using the anise plant's dry ripe fruits. Anise is a core essential oil for addressing digestive and respiratory imbalances. It is prized for its ability to clear respiratory congestion and relieve digestive stagnation or excess gas.

SOURCE COUNTRIES: Egypt and Spain

CORE COMPONENTS: Phenylpropanoid, trans-anethole

SAFETY: Due to the trans-anethole content and its estrogen-like activity, anise is contraindicated during pregnancy or breastfeeding or with individuals who have endometriosis or estrogen-dependent cancers.

CONSERVATION: Not defined

BLENDING WITH ANISE

AROMA: Sweet licorice-like, spicy, warm

SYSTEM AFFINITIES: Digestive, respiratory

BLENDS WELL WITH: Bergamot Mint, Cardamom, Celery Seed, Cinnamon Leaf, Clary Sage, Cypress, Sweet Fennel, Fingerroot, Geranium, Ginger, Lavender, Lemon, Neroli, Niaouli, Rose, Thyme ct. thymol

POTENTIAL SUBSTITUTIONS: Sweet Fennel, Thyme ct. thymol

THERAPEUTIC APPLICATIONS

INDICATIONS	METHOD OF APPLICATION	PAIRS WELL WITH
Digestive system: Upset stomach, gas, indigestion, nausea, bloating	Body oil for the stomach, personal inhaler	Cardamom, Celery Seed, Cinnamon Leaf, Clary Sage, Sweet Fennel, Fingerroot, Ginger, Lavender, Lemon, Thyme ct. thymol
Respiratory system: Respiratory congestion in lungs, bronchitis, spasmodic coughing, difficulty expelling excess mucus from nose	Chest salve, chest oil, diffusion, steam inhalation	Cardamom, Cinnamon Leaf, Clary Sage, Cypress, Fingerroot, Niaouli, Thyme ct. thymol
Reproductive system: Painful menstruation, menstrual cramping	Abdominal massage oil, unscented cream or lotion	Clary Sage, Sweet Fennel, Geranium, Lavender, Neroli, Rose
Psyche/emotions: Frigidity, difficulty processing what is happening in one's life, lack of creativity, emotional stagnation	Personal inhaler, diffuser, roll-on	Bergamot Mint, Cardamom, Celery Seed, Cinnamon Leaf, Clary Sage, Cypress, Sweet Fennel, Geranium, Lavender, Lemon, Neroli, Rose

SWEET BASIL CT. LINALOOL

Ahhh . . . beloved basil! **Sweet Basil** (*Ocimum basilicum*, Lamiaceae) essential oil is steam distilled using the leaves and flowering tops of the herb. This sweet basil, however, has a surprisingly different aroma than the basil used to make pesto. Rich in the calming aromatic component linalool, this basil calms and soothes digestive upsets, relieves cramps—be they digestive or menstrual—and reduces pain.

SOURCE COUNTRY: France

CORE COMPONENTS: Linalool, 1,8 cineole, eugenol, methyl cinnamate, β-caryophyllene, *a*-cubebene

SAFETY: No known contraindications or cautions

CONSERVATION: Least concern

BLENDING WITH BASIL CT. LINALOOL

AROMA: Sweet, spicy, fresh

SYSTEM AFFINITIES: Digestive, musculoskeletal, reproductive

BLENDS WELL WITH: Black Pepper, Cardamom, Clary Sage, Coriander Seed, Cypress, Sweet Fennel, Geranium, Ginger, Grapefruit, Jasmine, Juniper Berry, Lemon, Sweet Marjoram, Niaouli, Nutmeg, Sweet Orange, Palmarosa, Scots Pine, Pink Pepper, Rosemary ct. verbenone, Ylang Ylang

POTENTIAL SUBSTITUTIONS: Black Pepper + Lemon, Ginger, Clary Sage

THERAPEUTIC APPLICATIONS

INDICATIONS	METHOD OF APPLICATION	PAIRS WELL WITH
Digestive system: Upset stomach, excess gas, sluggish digestion	Abdominal massage oil, personal inhaler	Black Pepper, Coriander Seed, Sweet Fennel, Ginger, Sweet Marjoram, Nutmeg, Sweet Orange, Pink Pepper
Musculoskeletal system: Muscular tension caused by stress	Body oil for area of tension (e.g., neck and shoulders)	Black Pepper, Coriander Seed, Ginger, Juniper Berry, Sweet Marjoram, Ylang Ylang
Reproductive system: Menstrual cramps, painful menstruation, PMS (premenstrual syndrome)	Abdominal massage oil, personal inhaler	Black Pepper, Cardamom, Clary Sage, Coriander Seed, Sweet Fennel, Ginger, Jasmine, Sweet Marjoram, Nutmeg, Sweet Orange, Ylang Ylang
Psyche/emotions: Anxiety, mental fog, stress and stress-related conditions, e.g., headaches, upset stomach	Personal inhaler, diffusion, aromatic spritzer	Black Pepper, Cardamom, Clary Sage, Coriander Seed, Cypress, Sweet Fennel, Geranium, Ginger, Grapefruit, Jasmine, Juniper Berry, Lemon, Sweet Marjoram, Niaouli, Nutmeg, Sweet Orange, Palmarosa, Scots Pine, Pink Pepper, Rosemary ct. verbenone, Ylang Ylang

BERGAMOT

DIGESTIVE SYSTEM

Bergamot (*Citrus bergamia*, Rutaceae) essential oil can be distilled or expressed using the zest of the bergamot fruit. The bergamot tree is native to southern Italy, where the best bergamot essential oil is to be found. There are few essential oils that shine like bergamot in the realm of emotions. Bergamot both calms and soothes during times of stress while also supporting a balanced energy flow to keep you vibrant and motivated. Bergamot is uplifting and calming depending on what you blend with it. Clary sage and bergamot together would tend to be calming, whereas bergamot with eucalyptus would be stimulating.

SOURCE COUNTRIES: Southern Italy (Calabria), Ivory Coast, and Guinea

CORE COMPONENTS: D-limonene, linalool, and linalyl acetate

DERMAL CAUTION: Photosensitizer. The recommended dilution to avoid damage from sun is approximately one drop of essential oil per 1⅓ teaspoons (6.6 ml) of vegetable or other carrier oil, cream, or gel. We recommend avoiding application to the skin if going into the sun.

DERMAL ALERT: Bergamot has a shelf life of 1 to 2 years when stored correctly. Over time, bergamot, specifically its main component limonene, oxidizes. When this happens, there is an increase in the chance of dermal sensitization. Oxidized citrus essential oils such as bergamot should not be used in body care products for application to the skin. The essential oil can, however, be used for cleaning products.

CONSERVATION: Not yet defined

BLENDING WITH BERGAMOT

AROMA: Rich, exotic, fresh, sweet, sharp, citrus, becoming spicier after a time

SYSTEM AFFINITIES: Digestive

BLENDS WELL WITH: Angelica Root, Bergamot Mint, Cape Chamomile, Clary Sage, Coriander Seed, Frankincense, Geranium, Helichrysum, Jasmine, Lavender, Lemon, Lemongrass, Neroli, Peppermint, Petitgrain, Ylang Ylang

POTENTIAL SUBSTITUTIONS: Lemon + Grapefruit, Lavender + Sweet Orange + Grapefruit (equal parts), Clary Sage + Peppermint + Grapefruit

THERAPEUTIC APPLICATIONS

INDICATIONS	METHOD OF APPLICATION	PAIRS WELL WITH
Digestive system: Digestive upsets triggered by stress or exacerbated by stress	Personal inhaler, abdominal oil*, diffusion	Angelica Root, Bergamot Mint, Coriander Seed, Lavender, Lemon, Peppermint
Psyche/emotions: Anxiety, insomnia, emotional instability (mood swings), mild depression. Supports mental clarity, ability to focus, and memory. Reduces irritability	Bath in the evening*, personal inhaler, diffuser, roller ball* *Note: Refer to safety info above.	Angelica Root, Bergamot Mint, Cape Chamomile, Clary Sage, Coriander Seed, Frankincense, Geranium, Helichrysum, Jasmine, Lavender, Lemon, Lemongrass, Neroli, Peppermint, Petitgrain, Ylang Ylang

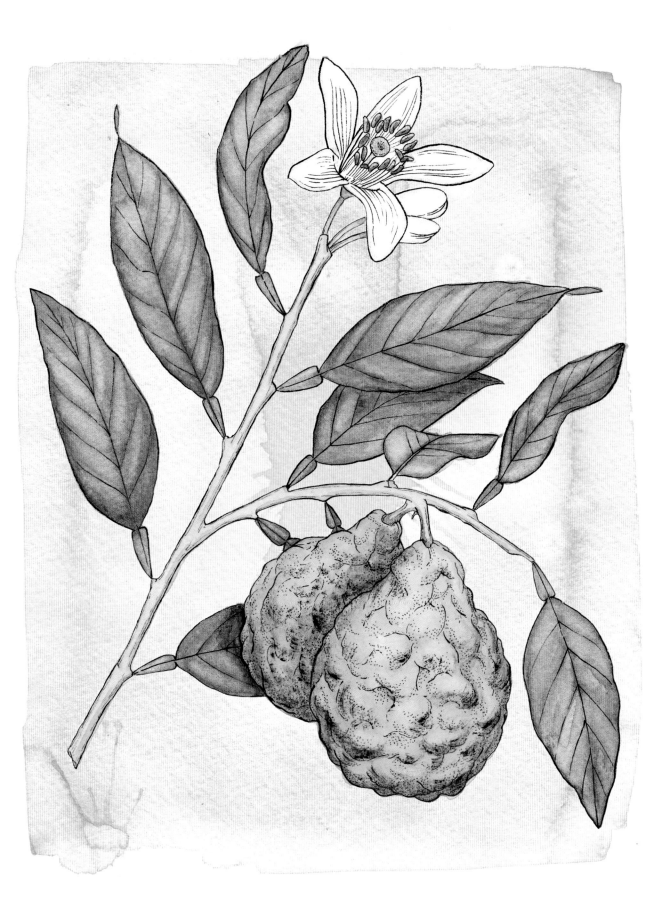

CARDAMOM

A native to Southern India, **Cardamom** (*Elettaria cardamomum*, Zingiberaceae) essential oil is steam distilled using the dried powdered seeds. Cardamom essential oil is a delicious essential oil for the digestive system. Not only does it support healthy digestion, it can help remove stagnation and eliminate painful gas. In other words, it can help you eliminate waste from the digestive system.

SOURCE COUNTRIES: Sri Lanka, Ceylon, and Guatemala

CORE COMPONENTS: 1,8 cineole, α-terpinyl acetate, limonene, linalyl acetate, sabinene

SAFETY FOR INFANTS/YOUNG CHILDREN: Do not apply to or near the face of infants or young children. Do not distill into nose/nasal cavity of infants or young children (e.g., with a nasal spray).

CONSERVATION: Not defined

BLENDING WITH CARDAMOM

AROMA: Spicy, warm, balsamic, sweet, penetrating, pungent

SYSTEM AFFINITIES: Digestive, respiratory

BLENDS WELL WITH: Bergamot, Black Pepper, Cinnamon Leaf, Clove Bud, Blue Gum Eucalyptus, Sweet Fennel, Laurel, Lemon, Green Myrtle, Scots Pine, Pink Pepper, Plai, Rose, Rosemary ct. cineole, Hemlock Spruce, Thyme ct. linalool or Thyme ct. thymol, Ylang Ylang

POTENTIAL SUBSTITUTIONS: Sweet Fennel

THERAPEUTIC APPLICATIONS

INDICATIONS	METHOD OF APPLICATION	PAIRS WELL WITH
Digestive system: Constipation, excess gas, colic, stomach upsets caused by emotional upsets or nervous conditions, nausea, heartburn, indigestion, sluggish digestion	Abdominal oil, personal inhaler, aromatic bath, roll-on	Black Pepper, Cinnamon Leaf, Clove Bud, Sweet Fennel, Lemon, Pink Pepper, Plai
Respiratory system: Bronchitis, excess coughing or tightness in lungs or chest caused by excess mucus, respiratory infection, damp congestion	Chest salve, chest oil, diffusion, steam inhalation, nebulizing diffuser	Eucalyptus, Sweet Fennel, Laurel, Lemon, Green Myrtle, Scots Pine, Pink Pepper, Plai, Rosemary ct. cineole, Spruce, Thyme ct. linalool or Thyme ct. thymol
Psyche/emotions: Anxiety, mild depression, poor concentration, lack of vital energy, mental stress	Personal inhaler, aromatic bath, roll-on, diffuser	Bergamot, Black Pepper, Cinnamon Leaf, Jasmine Absolute, Rose, Hemlock Spruce, Ylang Ylang

ROMAN CHAMOMILE

Roman Chamomile (*Chamaemelum nobile* syn. *Anthemis nobilis*, Asteraceae). Unlike German chamomile, Roman chamomile is not blue. It is a powerful remedy for soothing inflamed conditions of the skin. With its sweet apple-like aroma, it pairs well with mandarin and lavender for a room diffuser or personal inhaler to relax, calm, and encourage a good night's sleep! It is also a powerful remedy for muscle spasms.

SOURCE COUNTRIES: Italy, France, United States, Hungary, Chile, and Germany

CORE CHEMICAL COMPONENTS: Mix of unique ester components with isobutyl angelate, 2-methylbutyl angelate, isoamyl angelate, and isobutyl butyrate

DERMAL CAUTION: The likelihood of chamomile preparations causing a contact allergy is low. However, people with known sensitivities to other members of the Asteraceae (Compositae) family (including ragweed, daisies, and chrysanthemums) may want to avoid topical application of chamomile or chamomile products.[11]

CONSERVATION: Least concern

BLENDING WITH ROMAN CHAMOMILE

AROMA: Sweet, fruity, apple-like, strong

SYSTEM AFFINITIES: Digestive, skin

BLENDS WELL WITH: Angelica Root, Carrot Seed, Clary Sage, German Chamomile, Katafray, Lavender, Sweet Marjoram, Mandarin, Melissa

POTENTIAL SUBSTITUTIONS: German Chamomile, Cape Chamomile, Lavender, Sweet Marjoram

THERAPEUTIC APPLICATIONS

INDICATIONS	METHOD OF APPLICATION	PAIRS WELL WITH
Digestive system: Stress-related digestive upset or indigestion, bloating, excess gas, stomach cramps	Abdominal oil, personal inhaler, diffuser	Angelica Root, Carrot Seed, German Chamomile, Lavender
Skin: Inflamed/itchy skin conditions, dermatitis, eczema, psoriasis, broken capillaries, acne, slow-healing wounds, razor burn	Facial oil, body oil, unscented cream or lotion, gel, roll-on	Carrot Seed, German Chamomile, Lavender, Sweet Marjoram, Melissa, Thyme ct. linalool
Musculoskeletal system: Spasms, cramps, muscle tension	Body oil, gel, unscented cream or lotion	Clary Sage, German Chamomile, Katafray, Lavender, Sweet Marjoram, Mandarin
Psyche/emotions: Anxiety, anger, agitation, stress-related conditions, insomnia, feelings of being overwhelmed, headache or migraine triggered by stress, hyperactivity in children	Personal inhaler, diffuser, nebulizing diffuser, aromatic spritzer, roll-on	Angelica Root, Carrot Seed, Clary Sage, German Chamomile, Katafray, Lavender, Sweet Marjoram, Mandarin, Melissa, Thyme ct. linalool

FINGERROOT

Fingerroot (*Boesenbergia rotunda*, Zingiberaceae) essential oil is steam distilled using the bright yellow rhizomes of the fingerroot plant. Fingerroot is a traditional medicine of Malaysia, Thailand, Indonesia, India, and China, where it has been used for its antimicrobial properties, its ability to reduce inflammation, and its effectiveness on a variety of digestive disorders. The fingerroot essential oil offers many similar properties and more. A beautiful oil to work with, it is simultaneously energizing and calming.

SOURCE COUNTRIES: Malaysia, Thailand, and Indonesia

CORE COMPONENTS: β-ocimene, 1,8 cineole, camphor, camphene, geraniol, guaiol

SAFETY: No known contraindications or cautions

CONSERVATION: Not yet assessed

BLENDING WITH FINGERROOT

AROMA: Warming, camphoraceous, slightly floral with a slight citrus note

SYSTEM AFFINITIES: Digestive, respiratory

BLENDS WELL WITH: Angelica Root, Basil ct. linalool, Black Pepper, Clary Sage, Copaiba, Sweet Fennel, Frankincense, Ginger, Lavender, Lemon, Lemongrass, Sweet Marjoram, Myrrh, Petitgrain, Hemlock Spruce, Vetiver

POTENTIAL SUBSTITUTIONS: Ginger, Black Pepper

THERAPEUTIC APPLICATIONS

INDICATIONS	METHOD OF APPLICATION	PAIRS WELL WITH
Digestive system: Sluggish digestion, upset stomach, constipation, nausea	Abdominal oil, personal inhaler	Angelica Root, Basil ct. linalool, Black Pepper, Sweet Fennel, Ginger, Lemon, Lemongrass, Sweet Marjoram, Myrrh, Petitgrain, Hemlock Spruce, Vetiver
Respiratory System: Sinus congestion, bronchitis, cold	Steam inhalation	Frankincense, Lemon, Sweet Marjoram, Hemlock Spruce
Psyche/emotions: Anxiety, tension, lack of inspiration, lack of focus, foggy thinking, lack of libido, inability to manifest creative dreams	Personal inhaler, diffuser, roll-on	Angelica Root, Basil ct. linalool, Black Pepper, Clary Sage, Copaiba, Sweet Fennel, Frankincense, Ginger, Lavender, Lemon, Lemongrass, Sweet Marjoram, Myrrh, Petitgrain, Hemlock Spruce, Vetiver

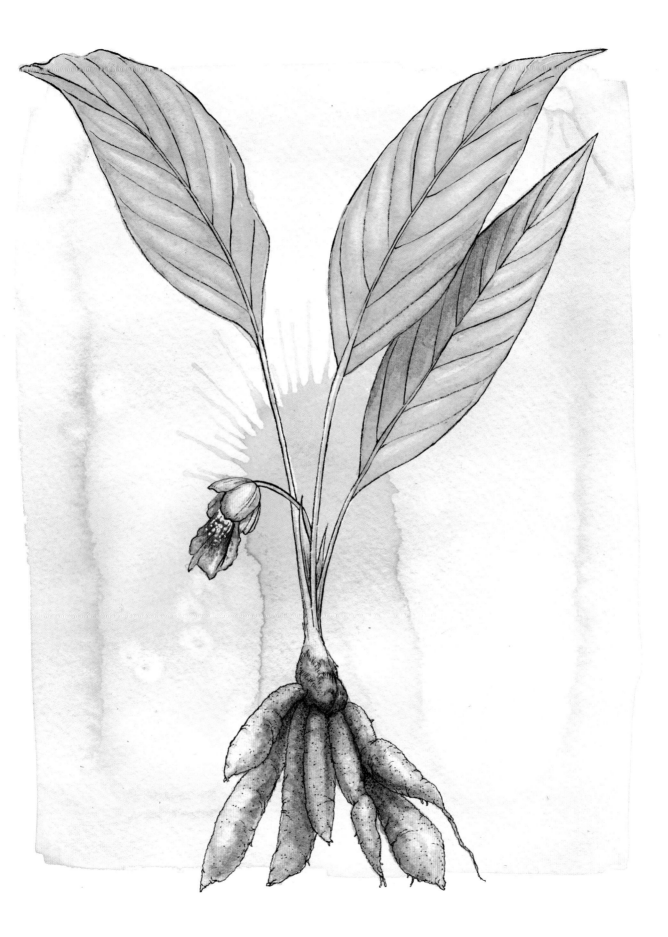

CORIANDER SEED

Coriander Seed (*Coriandrum sativum*, Apiaceae) essential oil is steam distilled using coriander seeds. Coriander is an annual and herbaceous plant native to southern Europe and western Mediterranean region. Coriander seed is often associated with digestive upsets triggered or made worse by stress.

SOURCE COUNTRIES: France, Italy, Morocco, and Russia

CORE COMPONENT: Linalool

SAFETY: No known contraindications or concerns

CONSERVATION: Not defined

BLENDING WITH CORIANDER SEED

AROMA: Sweet licorice-like, reminiscent of fennel

SYSTEM AFFINITIES: Digestive, respiratory, nervous

BLENDS WELL WITH: Bergamot, Black Pepper, Cape Chamomile, Carrot Seed, Roman Chamomile, Sweet Fennel, Ginger, Helichrysum, Katafray, Lavender, Sweet Marjoram, Mandarin, Neroli, Sweet Orange, Plai, Palmarosa, Pink Pepper, Rose, Valerian, Vetiver

POTENTIAL SUBSTITUTIONS: Lavender, Bergamot

THERAPEUTIC APPLICATIONS

INDICATIONS	METHOD OF APPLICATION	PAIRS WELL WITH
Digestive system: Indigestion, excess gas, constipation, nausea, stomach cramps, indigestion, poor appetite particularly when due to stress or feelings of being overwhelmed	Personal inhaler, abdominal oil, roll-on (for stress)	Black Pepper, Carrot Seed, Sweet Fennel, Ginger
Musculoskeletal system: General muscular aches and pains, muscular tension from stress or long hours at computer	Body oil, gel, salve, body butter	Black Pepper, Roman Chamomile, Ginger, Lavender, Sweet Marjoram, Pink Pepper, Plai, Vetiver
Psyche/emotions: Anxiety, chronic stress, mental fatigue or strain, nervous exhaustion, insomnia, feelings of being overwhelmed, study anxiety, excessive thinking or worry	Personal inhaler, body oil, diffuser, roll-on, nebulizing diffuser, aromatic bath	Bergamot, Cape Chamomile, Roman Chamomile, Ginger, Lavender, Sweet Marjoram, Mandarin, Neroli, Sweet Orange, Rose, Valerian, Vetiver

GINGER

Ginger (*Zingiber officinale*, Zingiberaceae) essential oil is steam distilled using dried or fresh ginger rhizome (root). Ginger has a long history of use as a fresh or dried herb and ginger essential oil. It shines in its ability to stimulate digestion, soothe excess gas or bloating, and support timely elimination.

SOURCE COUNTRIES: Sri Lanka, China, India, and Nigeria

CORE COMPONENTS: α-zingiberene, ar-curcumene, sabinene, (E,E)-α-farnesene, and β-sesquiphellandrene

DERMAL CAUTION: No known concerns or contraindications

CONSERVATION: Not defined

BLENDING WITH GINGER

AROMA: Spicy, warming

SYSTEM AFFINITIES: Digestive, musculoskeletal, respiratory

BLENDS WELL WITH: Angelica Root, Black Pepper, Cardamom, Clary Sage, Clove Bud, Coriander Seed, Sweet Fennel, Jasmine, Grapefruit, Rose, Lemongrass, Sweet Marjoram, Neroli, Plai, Ylang Ylang

POTENTIAL SUBSTITUTIONS: Black Pepper, Cardamom, Spearmint

THERAPEUTIC APPLICATIONS

INDICATIONS	METHOD OF APPLICATION	PAIRS WELL WITH
Digestive system: Stomachache, nausea, vomiting, morning sickness, excess gas, constipation, diarrhea, postoperative or drug-induced nausea, loss of appetite	Abdominal massage oil, personal inhaler, diffuser	Angelica Root, Black Pepper, Cardamom, Coriander Seed, Sweet Fennel, Grapefruit, Sweet Marjoram
Reproductive system: Lack of or reduced sex drive, impotence, menstrual cramps and pain, morning sickness (inhalation), dysmenorrhea	Body oil, personal inhaler, diffuser, abdominal oil	Clary Sage, Coriander Seed, Sweet Fennel, Jasmine Absolute, Grapefruit, Rose, Sweet Marjoram, Ylang Ylang
Musculoskeletal system: Muscular aches and pains, arthritis, sprains, rheumatism, joint pain and stiffness, warming	Cream or lotion, body oil, gel, salve	Black Pepper, Clary Sage, Clove Bud, Coriander Seed, Grapefruit, Lemongrass, Sweet Marjoram, May Chang, Plai
Psyche/emotions: Indecisiveness, confusion, frigidity, loss of motivation, burnout caused by chronic stress, lack of direction or focus, feelings of loneliness and resignation, poor memory, foggy thinking	Personal inhaler, body oil, diffuser, unscented cream or lotion	Angelica Root, Black Pepper, Cardamom, Clary Sage, Clove Bud, Coriander Seed, Sweet Fennel, Jasmine, Grapefruit, Rose, Lemongrass, Sweet Marjoram, Neroli, Plai, Ylang Ylang

GRAPEFRUIT

Grapefruit (*Citrus × paradise*, Rutaceae) essential oil is expeller pressed or distilled using the zest/rind of the grapefruit and is much beloved for its ability to uplift and inspire. Like all citrus oils, the aroma of grapefruit is used to relieve anxiety while uplifting one's energy and ability to focus. The compound nootkatone is responsible for the grapefruit's distinctive aroma. Traces of nootkatone have also been found in other citrus essential oils including bergamot, lemon, lime, orange, and tangerine.

SOURCE COUNTRIES: Israel, United States, and South Africa

CORE COMPONENT: D-limonene

SAFETY NOTE: Potential skin sensitizer if the oil is oxidized. Avoid older oils and store correctly.

CONSERVATION: Not defined

BLENDING WITH GRAPEFRUIT

AROMA: Fresh, citrusy, sweet

SYSTEM AFFINITY: Digestive

BLENDS WELL WITH: Bergamot, Bergamot Mint, Black Pepper, Cardamom, Cypress, Blue Gum Eucalyptus, Sweet Fennel, Geranium, Scots Pine, Jasmine Absolute, Juniper Berry, Lavender, Patchouli, Palmarosa, Peppermint, Rosemary ct. cineole, Ylang Ylang

POTENTIAL SUBSTITUTIONS: Lemon, Sweet Orange, Juniper Berry

THERAPEUTIC APPLICATIONS

INDICATIONS	METHOD OF APPLICATION	PAIRS WELL WITH
Digestive system: Constipation, sluggish digestion, digestion-related migraine	Abdominal oil, personal inhaler	Black Pepper, Cardamom, Sweet Fennel, Lemon, Peppermint
Reproductive system: PMS stress and/or tension	Personal inhaler, diffuser, roll-on	Cardamom, Sweet Fennel, Geranium, Grapefruit, Lavender, Lemon, Ylang Ylang
Skin: Oily/congested skin, cellulite, water retention, hair loss	Cleanser, unscented shampoo, salt scrub	Cypress, Geranium, Patchouli
Circulatory system: Sluggish circulation	Salt scrub	Blue Gum Eucalyptus, Grapefruit, Juniper Berry
Psyche/emotions: Mild depression, anxiety, stress, nervous exhaustion, agitation, irritability, stress-related conditions	Personal inhaler, body oil, diffuser, roll-on	Black Pepper, Cardamom, Jasmine Absolute, Ylang Ylang

SWEET ORANGE

Sweet Orange (*Citrus sinensis*, Rutaceae) essential oil is expressed or distilled using the zest of orange fruit. Sweet orange shines in its ability to uplift and yet calm emotions such as anxiety and stress. Its refreshing aroma also helps to relieve tension or stress-related health imbalances.

SOURCE COUNTRIES: Israel, United States, Spain, and Italy

CORE COMPONENTS: D-limonene

DERMAL ALERT: Sweet orange has a shelf life of 1 to 2 years when stored correctly. Over time, the main component of sweet orange (limonene) oxidizes. When this happens, there is an increase in the chance of dermal sensitization. Oxidized citrus essential oils should not be used in body care products for application to the skin. The essential oil can, however, be used for cleaning products.

CONSERVATION: Not defined

BLENDING WITH SWEET ORANGE

AROMA: Refreshing, citrusy, orange

SYSTEM AFFINITIES: Digestive

BLENDS WELL WITH: Clary Sage, Roman Chamomile, Himalayan Cedarwood, Coriander Seed, Frankincense, other citrus essential oils, Lavender, Sweet Marjoram, Neroli, Patchouli

POTENTIAL SUBSTITUTIONS: Mandarin, Lemon, Grapefruit, Bergamot

THERAPEUTIC APPLICATIONS

INDICATIONS	METHOD OF APPLICATION	PAIRS WELL WITH
Digestive system: Indigestion, nervous stomach, dyspepsia	Abdominal oil, personal inhaler, diffuser	Roman Chamomile, Coriander Seed, Lavender, Lemon, Sweet Marjoram
Psyche/emotions: Insomnia, anxiety, depression, agitation, restlessness, stress, irritability, depression	Personal inhaler, diffuser, nebulizing diffuser, roll-on, aromatic bath	Clary Sage, Roman Chamomile, Himalayan Cedarwood, Coriander Seed, Frankincense, other citrus essential oils, Lavender, Sweet Marjoram, Neroli, Patchouli

MANDARIN

Mandarin (*Citrus reticulata*, Rutaceae) essential oil is steam distilled or expressed using the peel/zest of the fruit. Mandarin is nurturing and warming, providing a sense of well-being. It's uplifting yet calming.

SOURCE COUNTRIES: Italy and Argentina

CORE COMPONENTS: D-limonene, γ-terpinene

SAFETY: No known contraindications or cautions. One of the safest oils to use for all ages.

DERMAL ALERT: Mandarin has a shelf life of 1 to 2 years when stored correctly. Over time, the main component of mandarin (limonene) oxidizes. When this happens, there is an increase in the chance of dermal sensitization. Oxidized citrus essential oils should not be used in body care products for application to the skin. The essential oil can, however, be used for cleaning products.

CONSERVATION: Not defined

BLENDING WITH MANDARIN

AROMA: Sweet, fresh, citrus

SYSTEM AFFINITIES: Digestive

BLENDS WELL WITH: Black Pepper, Roman Chamomile, Clary Sage, Coriander Seed, Geranium, Jasmine Absolute, Lavender, Lemon, Myrrh, Neroli, Sweet Orange, Palmarosa, Pink Pepper, Ylang Ylang

POTENTIAL SUBSTITUTIONS: Sweet Orange, Neroli, Lemon

THERAPEUTIC APPLICATIONS

INDICATIONS	METHOD OF APPLICATION	PAIRS WELL WITH
Digestive system: Stress-related digestive upset, dyspepsia, intestinal spasms. May gently stimulate appetite (especially after illness or depression)	Personal inhaler, abdominal oil, diffuser, nebulizing diffusor	Black Pepper, Roman Chamomile, Clary Sage, Coriander Seed, Lavender, Lemon, Sweet Orange, Pink Pepper
Reproductive system: PMS emotions or stress. Used during labor and delivery to ease tension	Personal inhaler, diffuser, roll-on, abdominal oil	Roman Chamomile, Clary Sage, Coriander Seed, Geranium, Lavender, Neroli, Sweet Orange, Ylang Ylang
Psyche/emotions: Tension, insomnia, nervous disorders, mild depression, hyperactivity in children, anxiety, stress, temper tantrums, anxiety	Personal inhaler, body oil, diffuser, nebulizing diffusor	Roman Chamomile, Clary Sage, Coriander Seed, Geranium, Jasmine Absolute, Lavender, Lemon, Myrrh, Neroli, Sweet Orange, Palmarosa, Ylang Ylang

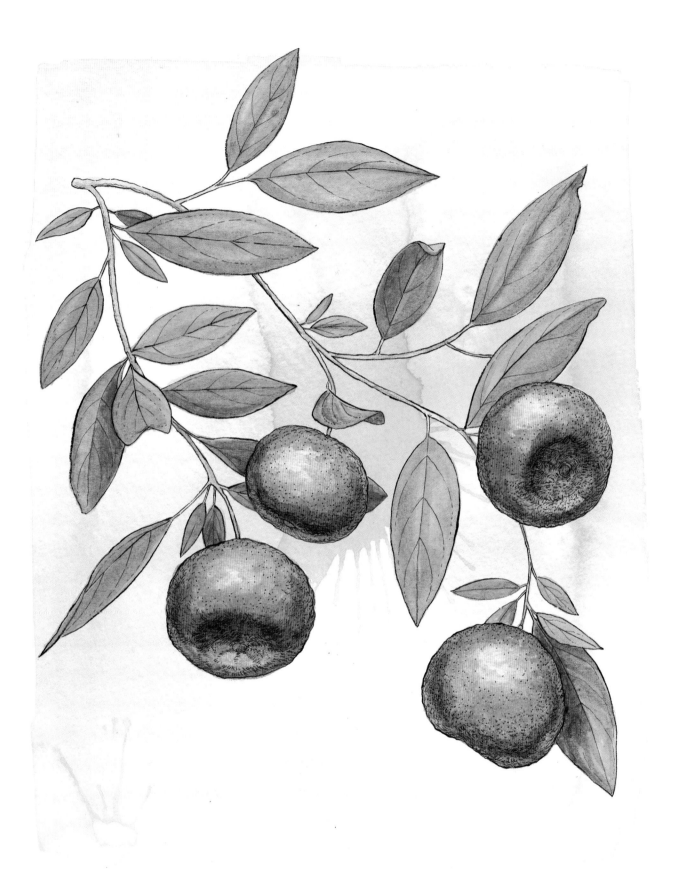

PINK PEPPER

Pink Pepper (*Schinus molle*, Anacardiaceae) essential oil is steam distilled using the dried pink pepper fruits. Although it has "pepper" in its name, it's unrelated to black pepper—though they do share some of the same characteristics. Pink pepper is a relative newcomer to the aromatherapy world. It is used for its pain-relieving activity for sore muscles and general aches and pains. And like black pepper, it supports healthy digestion and promotes circulation.

SOURCE COUNTRIES: Madagascar and Kenya

CORE COMPONENTS: β-caryophyllene, limonene, β-pinene, α-pinene

SAFETY: No known contraindications or cautions

CONSERVATION: Not yet assessed

BLENDING WITH PINK PEPPER

AROMA: Spicy, warming, slightly woody, light citrus

SYSTEM AFFINITIES: Musculoskeletal, digestive system

BLENDS WELL WITH: Black Pepper, Cardamom, Carrot Seed, Roman Chamomile, Cinnamon Leaf, Clove Bud, Sweet Fennel, Frankincense, Geranium, Ginger, Jasmine Absolute, Juniper Berry, Lavender, Patchouli, Rose, Vetiver, Ylang Ylang

POTENTIAL SUBSTITUTIONS: Black Pepper

THERAPEUTIC APPLICATIONS

INDICATIONS	METHOD OF APPLICATION	PAIRS WELL WITH
Digestive system: Indigestion, excess gas, sluggish digestion, lack of appetite	Personal inhaler, abdominal oil, diffuser	Black Pepper, Cardamom, Carrot Seed, Roman Chamomile, Cinnamon Leaf, Sweet Fennel, Ginger
Musculoskeletal system: Muscular aches and pains, rheumatism, muscle stiffness, arthritic pain	Body oil, gel, bath, salve	Black Pepper, Roman Chamomile, Clove Bud, Ginger, Juniper Berry, Lavender, Vetiver
Circulatory system: Poor circulation, Raynaud's syndrome, sensitivity to cold	Bath, salt scrub, hand or foot cream/lotion, body oil	Black Pepper, Cardamom, Carrot Seed, Ginger, Juniper Berry
Psyche/emotions: Mental fatigue, emotional coldness, apathy, low endurance, nervousness, weakness of will, loss of motivation, emotional exhaustion, indecisiveness	Personal inhaler, aromatic bath, diffuser, roll-on	Black Pepper, Cardamom, Roman Chamomile, Cinnamon Leaf, Frankincense, Geranium, Ginger, Jasmine Absolute, Lavender, Patchouli, Rose, Vetiver, Ylang Ylang

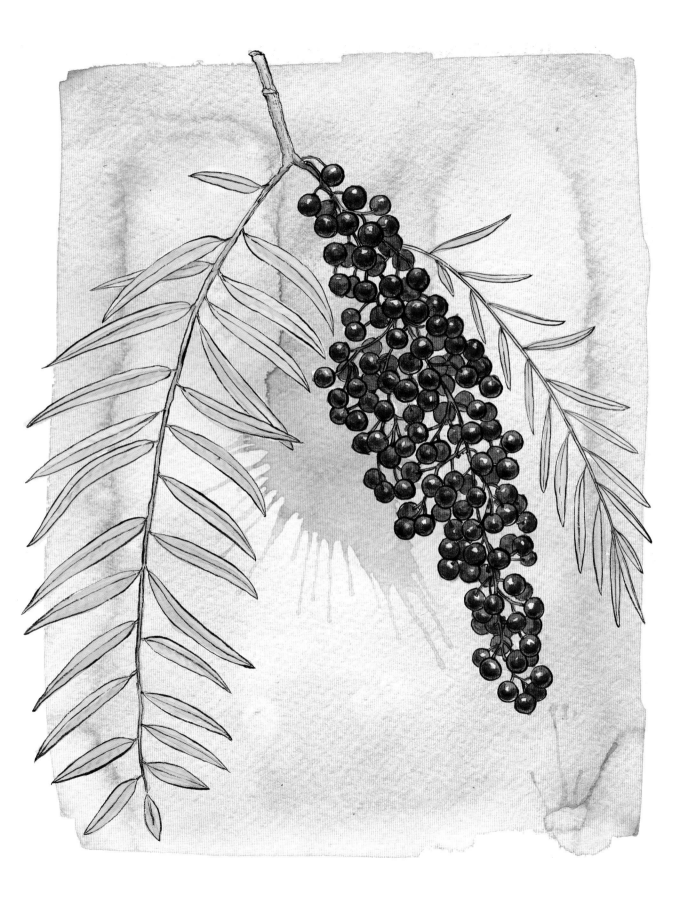

PEPPERMINT

Peppermint (*Mentha × piperita*, Lamiaceae) essential oil is steam distilled using the leaves. It is stimulating, invigorating, and uplifting. Peppermint essential oil is used to relieve digestive upsets, relieve nausea, reduce muscular aches and pains, and support the respiratory system during the cold and flu season.

SOURCE COUNTRIES: France, England, and United States

CORE COMPONENTS: Menthol, menthone

CONTRAINDICATION FOR INFANTS: Peppermint essential oil is contraindicated via any route for infants. Avoid application on or near the face of small children due to risk of respiratory spasm and arrest.

CONSERVATION: Least concern

BLENDING WITH PEPPERMINT

AROMA: Fresh, menthol, clean, cool, strong

SYSTEM AFFINITIES: Digestive, respiratory, musculoskeletal

BLENDS WELL WITH: Clary Sage, Coriander Seed, Blue Gum Eucalyptus, Sweet Fennel, Inula, Juniper Berry, Lavender, Laurel, Lemon, Sweet Marjoram

POTENTIAL SUBSTITUTIONS: Juniper Berry, Laurel

THERAPEUTIC APPLICATIONS

INDICATIONS	METHOD OF APPLICATION	PAIRS WELL WITH
Digestive system: Travel sickness, stomach upsets, cramping, gas with abdominal pain, nausea, irritable bowel syndrome	Abdominal oil, personal inhaler	Coriander Seed, Sweet Fennel, Lavender, Lemon, Sweet Marjoram
Musculoskeletal system: Muscular stiffness, aches and pains, tight muscles, rheumatism, fibromyalgia, sprains, arthritis, strains, plantar fasciitis, tendonitis, carpal tunnel syndrome, sciatica, bursitis	Body oil, salve, gel	Clary Sage, Coriander Seed, Blue Gum Eucalyptus, Juniper Berry, Lavender, Laurel, Lemon, Sweet Marjoram
Respiratory system: Bronchitis, sinusitis, spasmodic cough, head cold, common cold, congestion, flu	Personal inhaler, diffuser, nebulizing diffusor, chest salve, steam inhalation (use 1 drop only)	Blue Gum Eucalyptus, Inula, Laurel, Lemon, Sweet Marjoram, Niaouli, Rosemary ct. cineole or Rosemary ct. camphor, Thyme ct. thymol
Psyche/emotions: Fatigue, foggy thinking/cluttered mind, lethargy, apathy, mental fatigue, difficulty concentrating, tension headache, migraine, travel sickness, shock/trauma, inability to focus	Personal inhaler, roll-on, diffuser	Clary Sage, Coriander Seed, Blue Gum Eucalyptus, Juniper Berry, Lavender, Laurel, Lemon, Rosemary ct. cineole

CINNAMON LEAF

Cinnamon Leaf (*Cinnamomum verum*, Lauraceae) essential oil is steam distilled using the leaves of the cinnamon tree. Cinnamon leaf, with its spicy warming aroma, combined with ylang ylang and cardamom, creates an inspiring aphrodisiac body oil. Cinnamon leaf essential oil is also used for its pain relieving and broad-spectrum antimicrobial activity.

SOURCE COUNTRIES: Sri Lanka, Java, Madagascar, China

CORE COMPONENTS: Eugenol

DERMAL CAUTION: Moderate potential for skin sensitization

CONSERVATION: Not yet assessed

BLENDING WITH CINNAMON LEAF

AROMA: Pungent, spicy, warming, slightly woody, light

SYSTEM AFFINITIES: Digestive, respiratory

BLENDS WELL WITH: Bergamot Mint, Black Pepper, Cardamom, Clove Bud, Fingerroot, Frankincense, Ginger, Grapefruit, Lemon, Mandarin, Green Myrtle, Niaouli, Rose, Rosemary ct. cineole, Thyme ct. linalool or Thyme ct. thymol, Ylang Ylang

POTENTIAL SUBSTITUTIONS: Clove Bud

THERAPEUTIC APPLICATIONS

INDICATIONS	METHOD OF APPLICATION	PAIRS WELL WITH
Musculoskeletal system: Rheumatism, muscular spasm, muscular aches and pains	Body oil, salve, unscented cream	Bergamot Mint, Black Pepper, Clove Bud, Ginger, Grapefruit, Lemon
Respiratory system: Acute upper respiratory infections, cold, flu, bronchitis	Chest salve, steam inhalation (1 drop with other gentle essential oils such as lemon or cardamom), nebulizing diffuser, personal inhaler	Cardamom, Fingerroot, Lemon, Green Myrtle, Niaouli, Rosemary ct. cineole, Thyme ct. linalool, Thyme ct. thymol
Psyche/emotions: Exhaustion, weakness, depression, frigidity, lack of libido	Personal inhaler, diffuser, body oil, roll-on	Black Pepper, Cardamom, Clove Bud, Frankincense, Ginger, Grapefruit, Lemon, Mandarin, Rose, Ylang Ylang

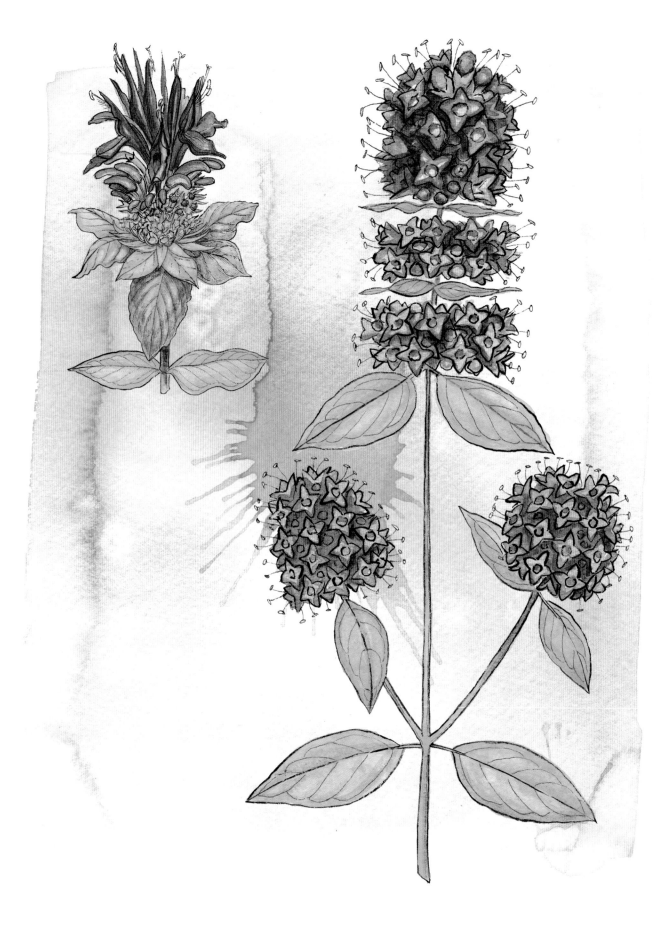

BERGAMOT MINT

Bergamot Mint (*Mentha citrate,* Lamiaceae) essential oil is steam distilled using the leaves of bergamot mint. Reminiscent of lavender with a splash of citrus, bergamot mint essential oil is both energizing and calming. With an affinity to the musculoskeletal system, bergamot mint essential oil can help relieve muscle aches and pains while also reducing tension and the physical or emotional manifestations of stress.

SOURCE COUNTRY: United States

CORE COMPONENTS: Linalool, linalyl acetate, geranyl acetate

SAFETY: No known contraindications or cautions

CONSERVATION: Not yet assessed

BLENDING WITH BERGAMOT MINT

AROMA: Soft, lemon-like yet floral, refreshing, slight citrus aroma

SYSTEM AFFINITIES: Muscular system

BLENDS WELL WITH: Basil ct. linalool, Bergamot, Black Pepper, Roman Chamomile, Clary Sage, Coriander Seed, Sweet Fennel, Geranium, Jasmine Absolute, Juniper Berry, Lavender, Lemon, Melissa, Sweet Orange, Petitgrain, Pink Pepper, Rose, Hemlock Spruce, Valerian, Ylang Ylang

POTENTIAL SUBSTITUTIONS: Lavender, Clary Sage, Coriander Seed

THERAPEUTIC APPLICATIONS

INDICATIONS	METHOD OF APPLICATION	PAIRS WELL WITH
Musculoskeletal system: Rheumatic pain, muscular aches and pains, muscular tension (e.g., from stress or long hours at the computer), muscular spasms or cramps	Body oil, gel, personal inhaler, unscented cream or lotion	Basil ct. linalool, Black Pepper, Roman Chamomile, Clary Sage, Coriander Seed, Juniper Berry, Lavender, Lemon, Pink Pepper
Psyche/emotions: Anxiety, chronic stress, mental fatigue or strain, nervous exhaustion, insomnia, stress and stress-related conditions, feelings of being overwhelmed, study anxiety, excessive thinking or worry stress, mental tension	Personal inhaler, aromatic bath, diffuser, aromatic spritzer	Basil ct. linalool, Bergamot, Black Pepper, Roman Chamomile, Clary Sage, Coriander Seed, Geranium, Jasmine Absolute, Lavender, Lemon, Melissa, Sweet Orange, Petitgrain, Rose, Valerian, Ylang Ylang

HIMALAYAN CEDARWOOD

Himalayan Cedarwood (*Cedrus deodara,* Pinaceae) essential oil is steam distilled using the wood. Himalayan cedarwood has many of the same qualities and benefits as Atlas cedar from Morocco, whose sustainability is in question. Its heavenly earthy wood sweet aroma soothes away tension while calming the mind. Himalayan cedarwood works well in body care products when a more "masculine" aroma is desired.

SOURCE COUNTRY: India

CORE COMPONENTS: β-himachalene, α-himachalene, (E)-α-atlantone

SAFETY: No known contraindications or cautions

CONSERVATION: Not yet assessed

BLENDING WITH HIMALAYAN CEDARWOOD

AROMA: Woody, balsamic, slightly sharp and smoky, balsamic. Subtle with a hint of spice

SYSTEM AFFINITIES: Skin, musculoskeletal

BLENDS WELL WITH: Bergamot, Bergamot Mint, Black Pepper, Calendula CO_2, Carrot Seed, Clary Sage, Clove Bud, Cypress, Frankincense, Ginger, Grapefruit, Lavender, Lemon, Lemongrass, Sweet Marjoram, Melissa, Myrrh, Palmarosa, Pinyon Pine, Rose, Vetiver, Ylang Ylang

POTENTIAL SUBSTITUTIONS: Red Cedar

THERAPEUTIC APPLICATIONS

INDICATIONS	METHOD OF APPLICATION	PAIRS WELL WITH
Musculoskeletal system: Muscular aches and pains, muscular tension	Body oil, unscented lotion, gel	Bergamot Mint, Black Pepper, Clary Sage, Clove Bud, Ginger, Lavender, Lemon, Lemongrass, Sweet Marjoram, Vetiver
Skin: Oily skin conditions, acne breakouts	Cleanser, gel, body butter	Calendula CO_2, Carrot Seed, Clary Sage, Cypress, Frankincense, Lavender, Lemon, Lemongrass, Melissa, Myrrh, Palmarosa, Rose
Psyche/emotions: Stress, anxiety, irritability, feelings of being overwhelmed, loss of center	Personal inhaler, aromatic bath, aromatic spritzer, roll-on	Bergamot, Bergamot Mint, Clary Sage, Frankincense, Grapefruit, Lavender, Lemon, Sweet Marjoram, Melissa, Myrrh, Pinyon Pine, Rose, Vetiver, Ylang Ylang

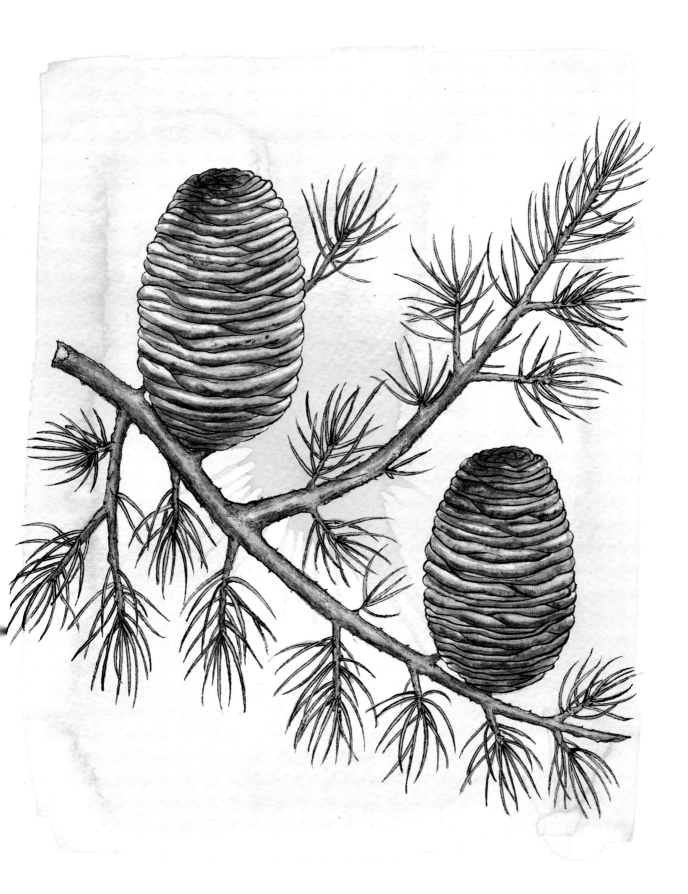

WINTERGREEN

Wintergreen (*Gaultheria procumbens*, Ericaceae) essential oil is steam distilled using wintergreen leaves. If you use an over-the-counter muscle aches-and-pain remedy, it most likely has wintergreen in it—or at least its active component, methyl salicylate. Wintergreen is a highly effective pain-relieving essential oil. It is powerful and needs to be used with care.

SOURCE COUNTRIES: China, India, Nepal, Sri Lanka, and the countries of North America

CORE COMPONENTS: Methyl salicylate

DERMAL CAUTION: Due to its ability to prevent blood clotting, wintergreen essential oil should NOT be used by those who have a bleeding or blood clot disorder, are on anticoagulant medication, are sensitive to aspirin or salicylates, or are just about to have major surgery. Pregnant or breastfeeding women should NOT use wintergreen. Young children are potentially at risk of Reye's Syndrome and should NOT use wintergreen essential oil internally or externally.

CONSERVATION: Not defined

BLENDING WITH WINTERGREEN

AROMA: Birch-like, fresh, penetrating

SYSTEM AFFINITIES: Circulatory, musculoskeletal, digestive

BLENDS WELL WITH: Blue Gum Eucalyptus, Laurel, Lavender, Lemon, Peppermint, Rosemary ct. verbenone

POTENTIAL SUBSTITUTIONS: Peppermint, Laurel

THERAPEUTIC APPLICATIONS

INDICATIONS	METHOD OF APPLICATION	PAIRS WELL WITH
Musculoskeletal system: Acute sharp pain, general aches and pains, muscular tension, tendonitis, muscle cramps, arthritis, tennis elbow, carpal tunnel syndrome, plantar fasciitis, rheumatic pain	Body oil, salve, gel, roll-on	Blue Gum Eucalyptus, Laurel, Lavender, Lemon, Peppermint, Rosemary ct. verbenone

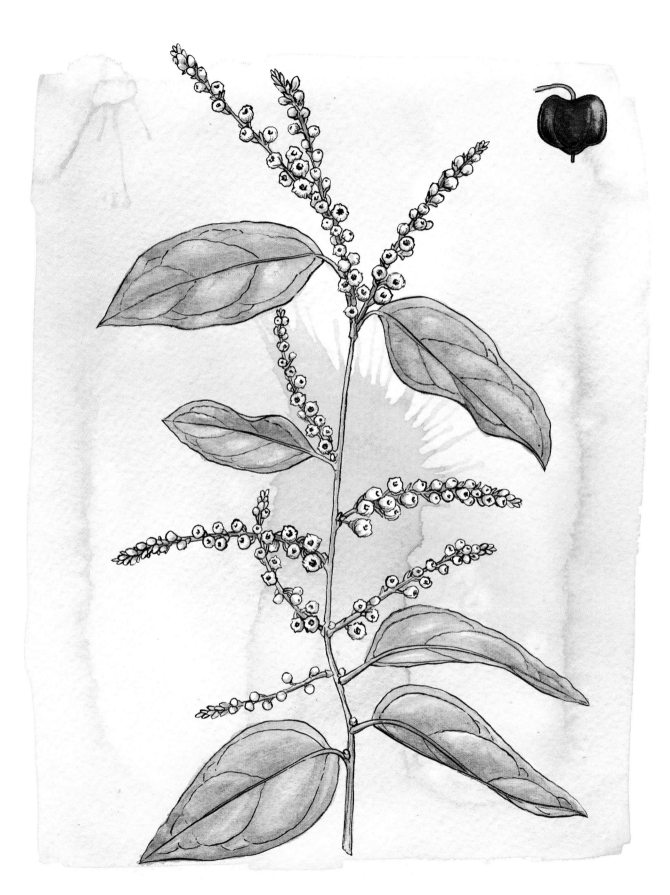

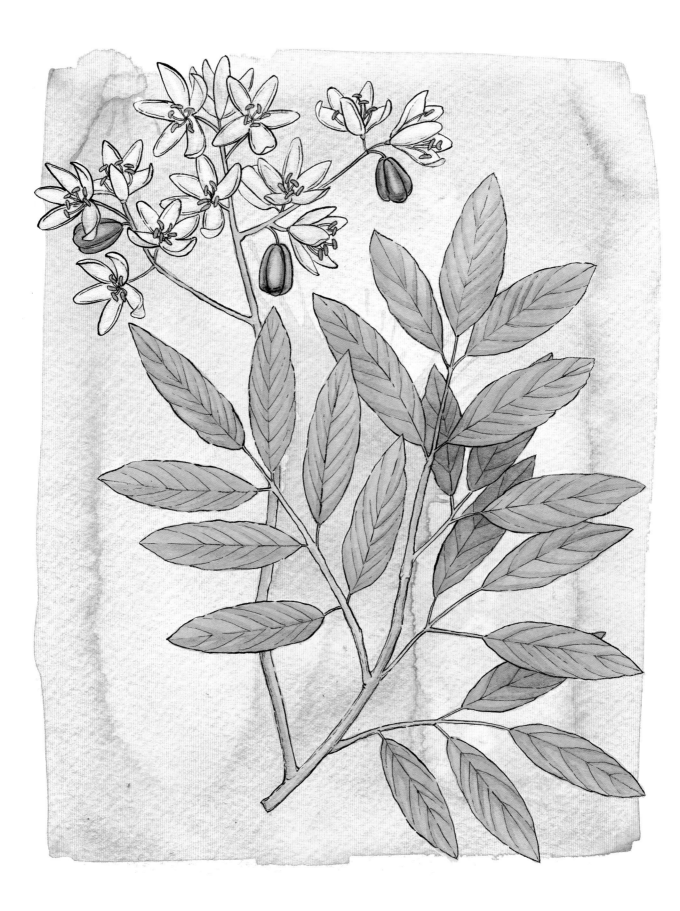

KATAFRAY

Katafray (*Cedrelopsis grevei*, Rutaceae) essential oil is steam distilled using the bark of the katafray tree. Prized for its ability to relieve muscular aches and pains, katafray also soothes and calms tension and irritability.

SOURCE COUNTRY: Madagascar

CORE COMPONENTS: Allo-aromadendrene, ishwarane, β-elemene

SAFETY: No known contraindications or cautions

CONSERVATION: Not yet assessed

BLENDING WITH KATAFRAY

AROMA: Woody with an earthy quality, balsamic, clear and penetrating

SYSTEM AFFINITIES: Musculoskeletal

BLENDS WELL WITH: Angelica Root, Basil ct. linalool, Black Pepper, Celery Seed, German Chamomile, Roman Chamomile, Clary Sage, Clove Bud, Frankincense, Geranium, Grapefruit, Lavender, Lemon, Sweet Orange, Petitgrain, Rose, Valerian, Wintergreen

POTENTIAL SUBSTITUTIONS: Basil ct. linalool, Lemongrass + Lavender, Black Pepper

THERAPEUTIC APPLICATIONS

INDICATIONS	METHOD OF APPLICATION	PAIRS WELL WITH
Musculoskeletal system: Rheumatism, muscle or joint stiffness, muscular aches and pains, muscle cramps or spasms	Body oil, salve, gel	Basil ct. linalool, Black Pepper, Roman Chamomile, Clove Bud, Grapefruit, Lavender, Lemon, Wintergreen
Psyche/emotions: Nervous tension, irritability, anxiety, nervousness, emotional ups and downs, feelings of being overwhelmed, low self-esteem, lack of focus	Personal inhaler, diffuser, roll-on	Angelica Root, Basil ct. linalool, Celery Seed, German Chamomile, Roman Chamomile, Clary Sage, Clove Bud, Frankincense, Geranium, Grapefruit, Lavender, Lemon, Sweet Orange, Rose

PLAI

Plai (*Zingiber cassumunar*, Zingiberaceae) essential oil is steam distilled using the fresh rhizomes of the plai plant. Plai is a newer essential oil to the aromatherapy world, but it makes its mark as an effective pain reliever.

SOURCE COUNTRY: Thailand

CORE COMPONENTS: Sabinene, γ-terpinene, α-terpinene, terpinen-4-ol

SAFETY: No known contraindications or cautions

CONSERVATION: Not yet assessed

BLENDING WITH PLAI

AROMA: Earthy, herbaceous

SYSTEM AFFINITIES: Musculoskeletal, respiratory

BLENDS WELL WITH: Angelica Root, Black Pepper, Cardamom, Himalayan Cedarwood, Roman Chamomile, Clary Sage, Copaiba, Coriander Seed, Sweet Fennel, Fingerroot, Ginger, Lemongrass, Sweet Marjoram, Melissa, Niaouli, Sweet Orange, Palmarosa, Petitgrain

POTENTIAL SUBSTITUTIONS: Blue Tansy, Sweet Marjoram

THERAPEUTIC APPLICATIONS

INDICATIONS	METHOD OF APPLICATION	PAIRS WELL WITH
Musculoskeletal system: Rheumatic pain, muscular aches and pains, arthritis, joint pain, cramps or spasms	Body oil, salve, unscented cream or lotion	Black Pepper, Himalayan Cedarwood, Roman Chamomile, Clary Sage, Coriander Seed, Ginger, Lemongrass, Sweet Marjoram
Respiratory system: Allergies, hay fever, asthma	Personal inhaler, nebulizing diffuser, diffuser	Cardamom, Fingerroot, Sweet Marjoram, Niaouli
Reproductive system: Menstrual cramps, painful menstruation (dysmenorrhea)	Abdominal massage	Clary Sage, Sweet Fennel, Sweet Marjoram
Psyche/emotions: Stress, anxiety, foggy thinking, confusion	Personal inhaler, roll-on	Angelica Root, Cardamom, Himalayan Cedarwood, Roman Chamomile, Clary Sage, Coriander Seed, Sweet Marjoram, Sweet Orange, Palmarosa, Petitgrain

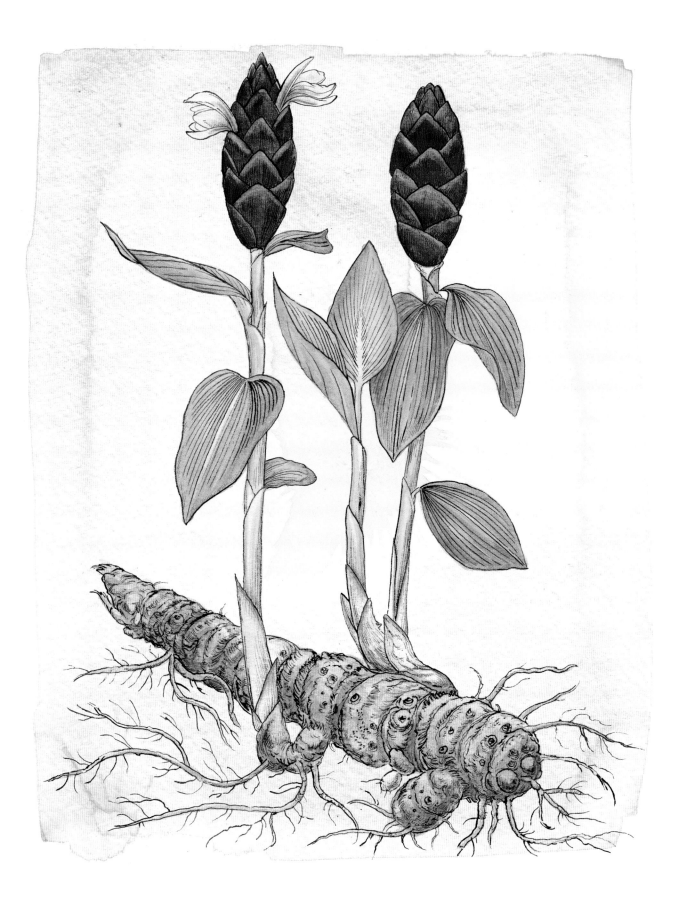

VETIVER

Vetiver (*Chrysopogon zizanioides* syn. *Vetiveria zizanioides*, Poaceae), also known as ruh khus, essential oil is steam distilled using the roots of vetiver grass. Vetiver essential oil can ground one in one's experience and life while relieving the stressors of the day. It provides a sense of focus when one is feeling overwhelmed.

SOURCE COUNTRIES: Haiti, Sri Lanka, and India

CORE COMPONENTS: Vetiver is one of the most complex essential oils; sesquiterpenols, sesquiterpenes, esters

DERMAL CAUTION: No known contraindications

CONSERVATION: Not defined

BLENDING WITH VETIVER

AROMA: Sweet, earthy, warm, woody, deep

SYSTEM AFFINITIES: Psyche/emotion, musculoskeletal

BLENDS WELL WITH: Bergamot, Cistus, Cypress, Fingerroot, Geranium, Ginger, Grapefruit, Lavender, Lemon, Lemongrass, Myrrh, Neroli, Patchouli, Petitgrain, Pink Pepper, Plai, Rose, Hemlock Spruce, Ylang Ylang

POTENTIAL SUBSTITUTIONS: Patchouli, Ginger, Cypress, Rose

THERAPEUTIC APPLICATIONS

INDICATIONS	METHOD OF APPLICATION	PAIRS WELL WITH
Musculoskeletal system: Muscular aches and pains, sprains, stiffness, muscle tension, arthritis, rheumatism	Body oil, gel, salve, body butter, unscented lotion	Ginger, Lavender, Lemon, Lemongrass, Pink Pepper, Plai
Circulatory system: Varicose veins, poor circulation	Body oil, salt scrub	Cistus, Cypress, Geranium, Ginger, Grapefruit, Lavender, Lemon, Lemongrass, Pink Pepper, Rose
Skin: Acne, inflamed conditions, oily skin, irritated skin. Preventative for stretch marks and wrinkles	Facial cleanser, unscented cream or lotion, salt scrub, body butter	Cistus, Cypress, Geranium, Lavender, Lemon, Lemongrass, Myrrh, Neroli, Patchouli, Petitgrain, Rose
Psyche/emotions: Physical and mental burnout, lack of confidence, anxiety, depression. Settles nerves before an ordeal (lecture, dentist)	Personal inhaler, aromatic bath, body butter	Bergamot, Cistus, Cypress, Fingerroot, Geranium, Ginger, Grapefruit, Lavender, Lemon, Lemongrass, Myrrh, Neroli, Patchouli, Petitgrain, Pink Pepper, Plai, Rose, Hemlock Spruce, Ylang Ylang

LAUREL

Laurel (*Laurus nobilis*, Lauraceae) essential oil is steam distilled using laurel tree leaves. It inspires and uplifts the spirit and increases focus and concentration. Laurel also has pain-relieving actions for sore muscles/ joints and expectorant traits for respiratory congestion.

SOURCE COUNTRIES: Morocco, France, and Croatia

CORE COMPONENTS: 1,8 cineole, sabinene, trans-sabinene hydrate

CAUTION FOR CHILDREN: Avoid application of 1,8 cineole-rich essential oils to the face or near the nose of infants and children. Use low dilutions (less than 1percent) with children between 3 and 7 years.

DERMAL APPLICATION CAUTION: Use caution when applying laurel essential oil to hypersensitive, diseased, or damaged skin, or on the skin of children under 2.

CONSERVATION: Least concern

BLENDING WITH LAUREL

AROMA: Sweet, fresh, slightly minty, camphoraceous

SYSTEM AFFINITIES: Respiratory, musculoskeletal

BLENDS WELL WITH: Basil ct. linalool, Bergamot Mint, Cape Chamomile, Cypress, Balsam Fir, Frankincense, Grapefruit, Himalayan Cedarwood, Inula, Juniper Berry, Lemon, Sweet Marjoram, Green Myrtle, Niaouli, Peppermint, Scots Pine

POTENTIAL SUBSTITUTIONS: Blue Gum Eucalyptus

THERAPEUTIC APPLICATIONS

INDICATIONS	METHOD OF APPLICATION	PAIRS WELL WITH
Musculoskeletal system: Strains, rheumatism, muscle or joint stiffness, muscular aches and pains, fibromyalgia, plantar fasciitis, carpal tunnel syndrome, arthritis, rheumatoid arthritis	Roll on, body (massage) oil, lotion, aromatic bath	Basil ct. linalool, Bergamot Mint, Grapefruit, Juniper Berry, Lemon, Sweet Marjoram, Peppermint, Scots Pine, Pinyon Pine, Plai, Rosemary (all chemotypes), Saro, Tea Tree, Vetiver, Wintergreen
Respiratory system: Bronchitis, colds, flu or influenza, viral infections	Steam inhalation, personal inhaler, chest salve, chest oil, aromatic baths	Cypress, Balsam Fir, Frankincense, Himalayan Cedarwood, Inula, Juniper Berry, Lemon, Sweet Marjoram, Green Myrtle, Niaouli, Peppermint, Scots Pine, Pinyon Pine, Rosemary ct. cineole, Saro, Tea Tree
Psyche/emotions: Nervous tension, exhaustion, poor concentration or memory recall, depression	Personal inhaler, abdominal oil, diffusion	Basil ct. linalool, Bergamot Mint, Cape Chamomile, Cypress, Balsam Fir, Frankincense, Grapefruit, Himalayan Cedarwood, Juniper Berry, Lemon, Sweet Marjoram, Scots Pine, Pinyon Pine, Vetiver

LEMONGRASS

West Indian **Lemongrass** (*Cymbopogon flexuosus*, Poaceae) or East Indian Lemongrass (*Cymbopogon citratus*) essential oils are steam distilled using the grass. Chemically very similar, both essential oils are used to relieve muscular aches and pains while also calming stress and relieving tension.

SOURCE COUNTRIES: Nepal and countries of the West Indies

CORE COMPONENTS: Neral and geranial, geraniol, *Cymbopogon flexuosus* also contains β-myrcene

DERMAL CAUTION: Use caution when applying lemongrass essential oil to hypersensitive, diseased, or damaged skin. Always dilute in carrier oil for application to the skin. If you are going to clean with lemongrass in warm water, use gloves!

CONSERVATION: Not defined

BLENDING WITH LEMONGRASS

AROMA: Lemony, strong, herbaceous

SYSTEM AFFINITIES: Musculoskeletal

BLENDS WELL WITH: Basil ct. linalool, Bergamot Mint, Black Pepper, Clary Sage, Copaiba, Cypress, Himalayan Cedarwood, Frankincense, Geranium, Ginger, Jasmine Absolute, Lavender, Palmarosa, Patchouli, Peppermint, Pink Pepper, Plai, Ylang Ylang

POTENTIAL SUBSTITUTIONS: Lemon, Palmarosa

THERAPEUTIC APPLICATIONS

INDICATIONS	METHOD OF APPLICATION	PAIRS WELL WITH
Musculoskeletal system: Muscular aches and pains, tired and sore muscles, sprains, bruises, weakness of connective tissue, pain in joints, muscle weakness	Gel, unscented cream or lotion, salve, body oil	Basil ct. linalool, Bergamot Mint, Black Pepper, Ginger, Lavender, Peppermint, Pink Pepper, Plai
Psyche/emotions: Fatigue, grieving process, strengthening during weak emotional period, transition, release work	Personal inhaler, salt inhaler	Bergamot Mint, Basil ct. linalool, Clary Sage, Copaiba, Himalayan Cedarwood, Frankincense, Geranium, Ginger, Jasmine Absolute, Lavender, Palmarosa, Patchouli, Ylang Ylang

CLARY SAGE

Clary Sage (*Salvia sclarea*, Lamiaceae) essential oil is steam distilled using the flowering tops of the clary sage plant. Clary sage has a powerful affinity with the feminine and is used for premenstrual tension or mood swings, menstrual cramps, and irregular menstrual cycles. It is also a powerful essential oil for women going through perimenopause, providing strength and a sense of balance. Its pungent floral aroma inspires creativity, acceptance, and joy.

SOURCE COUNTRIES: France, Germany, and Russia

CORE COMPONENTS: Linalool and linalyl acetate

SAFETY: No known contraindications or cautions

CONSERVATION: Least concern

BLENDING WITH CLARY SAGE

AROMA: Sweet, nutty, floral, earthy

SYSTEM AFFINITIES: Reproductive, musculoskeletal

BLENDS WELL WITH: Basil ct. linalool, Bergamot, Bergamot Mint, Black Pepper, Cardamom, German Chamomile, Sweet Fennel, Geranium, Ginger, Goldenrod, Grapefruit, Lavender, Mandarin, Sweet Marjoram, Peppermint, Pink Pepper, Plai, Rose, Valerian, Vetiver

POTENTIAL SUBSTITUTIONS: Lavender, Sweet Fennel, Geranium

THERAPEUTIC APPLICATIONS

INDICATIONS	METHOD OF APPLICATION	PAIRS WELL WITH
Reproductive system: Menstrual cycle irregularities, PMS and related upsets, cramps, menopause, childbirth/labor, painful menstruation, hot flashes, night sweats, hormonal irritability and imbalance	Abdominal massage oil, personal inhaler, diffusion, baths, hydrosol spray	Bergamot, Sweet Fennel, Peppermint, Geranium, Lavender, Sweet Orange, Ylang Ylang, Petitgrain, Rose, Vetiver
Musculoskeletal system: Aches and pains, arthritis, rheumatism, muscle spasms or cramps, sciatica, carpal tunnel syndrome, plantar fasciitis	Body oil, salve, cream/lotion	Bergamot, Peppermint, Lavender, Sweet Orange, Vetiver
Psyche/emotions: Irritability, anger, mental fatigue, anxiety, insomnia, mild depression, mild postnatal depression, exhaustion from overwork	Personal inhaler, abdominal oil, diffusion	Basil ct. linalool, Bergamot, Bergamot Mint, Black Pepper, Cardamom, German Chamomile, Sweet Fennel, Geranium, Ginger, Goldenrod, Grapefruit, Lavender, Mandarin, Sweet Marjoram, Peppermint, Pink Pepper, Plai, Rose, Valerian, Vetiver

JASMINE ABSOLUTE

Known as the Queen of Night, **Jasmine** (*Jasminum grandiflorum*, Oleaceae) absolute is solvent extracted using jasmine flowers picked at night. The oil is dark orange or brown. This intoxicating absolute not only lifts and inspires the spirits, it is also much admired as an aphrodisiac.

SOURCE COUNTRY: France

CORE COMPONENTS: Benzyl acetate, benzyl benzoate

DERMAL CAUTION: Moderate risk of skin sensitization

CONSERVATION: Not defined

BLENDING WITH JASMINE ABSOLUTE

AROMA: Rich, floral, fruity, heady, exotic

SYSTEM AFFINITIES: Psyche/emotions, reproductive

BLENDS WELL WITH: Angelica Root, Bergamot, Black Pepper, Cypress, Grapefruit, Mandarin, Sweet Orange, Palmarosa, Patchouli, Pink Pepper, Plai, Rose, Ylang Ylang

POTENTIAL SUBSTITUTIONS: Ylang Ylang, Neroli

THERAPEUTIC APPLICATIONS

INDICATIONS	METHOD OF APPLICATION	PAIRS WELL WITH
Reproductive system: Frigidity and impotence, uterine pain, postpartum depression, PMS, dysmenorrhea (painful menstruation). Facilitates childbirth/delivery	Personal inhaler, abdominal oil, body oil	Angelica Root, Bergamot, Black Pepper, Cypress, Grapefruit, Mandarin, Sweet Orange, Pink Pepper, Rose, Ylang Ylang
Psyche/emotions: Depression, nervous exhaustion, lack of confidence, lethargy, anxiety, obsessive thinking, tension, agitation, insomnia, loss or lack of libido	Personal inhaler, roll-on, body oil	Angelica Root, Bergamot, Black Pepper, Cypress, Grapefruit, Mandarin, Sweet Orange, Patchouli, Pink Pepper, Rose, Ylang Ylang

YLANG YLANG

Ylang Ylang (*Cananga odorata*, Annonaceae) essential oil is steam distilled using the flowers of the ylang ylang tree. Ylang ylang is a perennial tropical aromatic tree that originated in the Philippines and has now spread throughout tropical Asia. The essential oil is sometimes referred to as "poor man's jasmine," and indeed it shares many of the same properties and abilities. Ylang ylang is best known for its aphrodisiac qualities, along with being euphoric.

SOURCE COUNTRIES: Reunion Islands, Comoros, and Madagascar

CORE COMPONENTS: There are three types of ylang ylang essential oils available: Ylang Ylang Extra or Extra Superior is rich in linalool and benzyl acetate; Ylang Ylang #2 is rich in linalool, benzyl acetate, geranyl acetate; and Ylang Ylang #3 is rich in linalool, benzyl acetate, geranyl acetate, germacrene-D, benzyl benzoate

DERMAL CAUTION: Use caution when applying to hypersensitive, diseased, or damaged skin

CAUTION FOR CHILDREN AND INFANTS: Avoid dermal application of ylang ylang essential oil to children under 2 years of age.

CONSERVATION: Not defined

BLENDING WITH YLANG YLANG

AROMA: Warm, exotic, sweet, heavy, sensual

SYSTEM AFFINITIES: Psyche/emotions

BLENDS WELL WITH: Basil ct. linalool, Bergamot, Bergamot Mint, Cardamom, Clary Sage, Cinnamon Leaf, Frankincense, Geranium, Ginger, Jasmine Absolute, Lavender, Mandarin, Sweet Orange, Palmarosa, Patchouli, Petitgrain, Rose

POTENTIAL SUBSTITUTIONS: Neroli, Cinnamon Leaf, Patchouli

THERAPEUTIC APPLICATIONS

INDICATIONS	METHOD OF APPLICATION	PAIRS WELL WITH
Reproductive system: PMS, low self-esteem, painful menstruation, low libido, PMT (premenstrual tension)	Personal inhaler, diffuser, body oil, abdominal oil	Basil ct. linalool, Clary Sage, Geranium, Ginger, Jasmine Absolute, Lavender, Mandarin, Sweet Orange, Patchouli, Petitgrain, Rose
Psyche/emotions: Anxiety, anger, bereavement, separation, post-traumatic stress syndrome, nervous tension or depression, frigidity, high blood pressure from stress. An antidepressant; very calming	Personal inhaler, diffuser, roll-on	Basil ct. linalool, Bergamot, Bergamot Mint, Cardamom, Clary Sage, Cinnamon Leaf, Frankincense, Geranium, Ginger, Jasmine Absolute, Lavender, Mandarin, Sweet Orange, Palmarosa, Patchouli, Petitgrain, Rose

AMMI

Ammi (*Ammi visnaga*, Apiaceae) essential oil is steam distilled using the seeds from the Ammi umbels. Highly prized for its ability to relax and relieve spasm or constriction of the respiratory system (e.g., spasmodic coughs or asthma).

SOURCE COUNTRY: Morocco

CORE COMPONENTS: Esters (2-methylbutyl isobutyrate, 2-methylbutyl 2-methylbutanoate)

DERMAL CAUTION: Potentially phototoxic

CONSERVATION: Not yet assessed

BLENDING WITH AMMI

AROMA: Earthy, herbaceous

SYSTEM AFFINITIES: Respiratory system

BLENDS WELL WITH: Hyssop decumbens, Lavender, Thyme ct. linalool

POTENTIAL SUBSTITUTIONS: Green Myrtle

THERAPEUTIC APPLICATIONS

INDICATIONS	METHOD OF APPLICATION	BLENDS WELL WITH
Respiratory system: Asthma, spasmodic coughing	Gel, unscented cream or lotion, salve, aromatic baths,	Hyssop decumbens, Lavender, Thyme ct. linalool

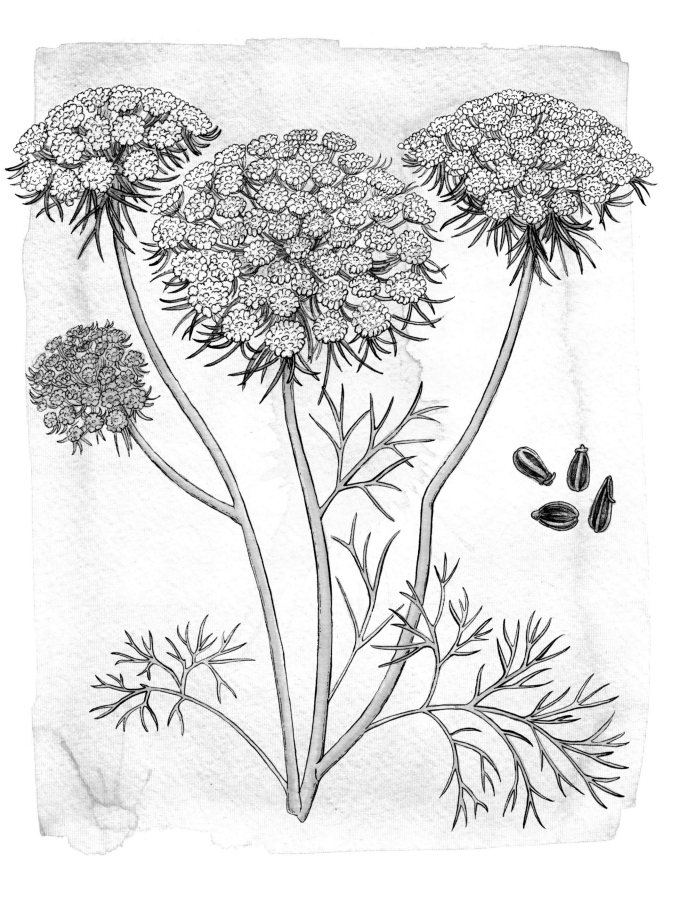

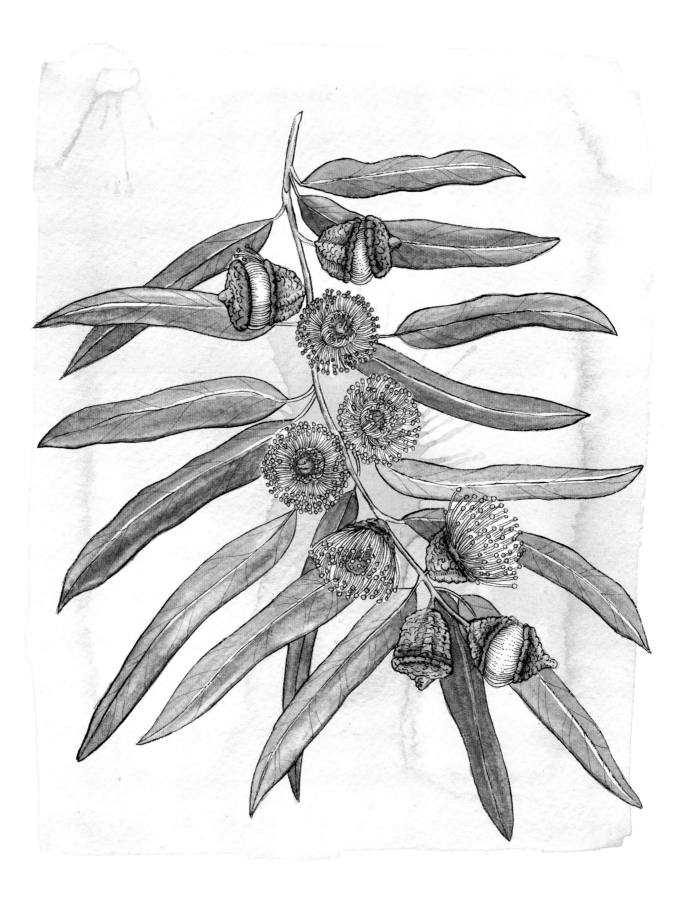

BLUE GUM EUCALYPTUS

Indigenous to Australia, **Blue Gum Eucalyptus** (*Eucalyptus globulus*, Myrtaceae) essential oil is steam distilled using leaves and mature branches of the eucalyptus tree. Its strong affinity with the respiratory system makes it the go-to essential oil for respiratory congestion. Eucalyptus is also beneficial for relieving muscular aches and pains and offers an uplifting and energizing aroma.

SOURCE COUNTRIES: South Africa and Australia

CORE COMPONENTS: 1,8 cineole

CAUTION FOR CHILDREN: Avoid application of 1,8 cineole–rich essential oils to the face or near the nose of infants and children under the age of 5 years. Do not instill 1,8 cineole-rich essential oils into the nose of infants or children. Use low dilutions (less than 1percent) with children aged 3 to 7 years.

CONSERVATION: Not defined

BLENDING WITH EUCALYPTUS

AROMA: Strong, camphor-like, balsamic, fresh

SYSTEM AFFINITIES: Respiratory

BLENDS WELL WITH: Cardamom, Laurel, Lavender, Lemon, Green Myrtle, Plai, Peppermint, Scots Pine, Rosemary ct. cineole, Hemlock Spruce

POTENTIAL SUBSTITUTIONS: Rosemary ct. cineole, Laurel, Niaouli

THERAPEUTIC APPLICATIONS

INDICATIONS	METHOD OF APPLICATION	PAIRS WELL WITH
Respiratory system: Bronchitis, sinusitis, rhinitis, nasal congestion, coughs, cold, flu, pertussis, bronchial mucus congestion	Steam inhalation, personal inhaler, chest salve, chest oil, aromatic baths	
Musculoskeletal system: Muscular aches and pains, arthritis, rheumatism, plantar fasciitis, sprains	Gel, body oil, salve	Cardamom, Laurel, Peppermint, Plai, Rosemary ct. cineole
Psyche/emotions: Foggy thinking, sluggishness, emotional heaviness, lack of energy/vibrancy	Personal inhaler, roll-on, diffuser, nebulizing diffuser	Cardamom, Laurel, Lemon, Lavender, Peppermint, Rosemary ct. cineole

BALSAM FIR

Balsam Fir (*Abies balsamea*, Pinaceae) essential oil is steam distilled using needles and young twigs of the fir tree. This beautiful fir is reminiscent of a forest walk and naturally deepens and expands the breath, reducing stress or anxiety while also gently energizing and uplifting.

SOURCE COUNTRY: Canada

CORE COMPONENTS: β-pinene, bornyl acetate, α-pinene, delta-3-carene, β-phellandrene, d-limonene

DERMAL CAUTION: Potential skin sensitizer if the oil is oxidized. Avoid older oils and store correctly.

CONSERVATION: Not yet assessed

BLENDING WITH BALSAM FIR

AROMA: Fresh, coniferous, pine-like, reminiscent of the forest

SYSTEM AFFINITY: Respiratory

BLENDS WELL WITH: Bergamot, Black Pepper, Blue Gum Eucalyptus, Frankincense, Juniper Berry, Lavender, Lemon, Niaouli, Peppermint, Scots Pine, Rosemary ct. cineole or Rosemary ct. camphor, Hemlock Spruce, Tea Tree, Thyme ct. linalool or Thyme ct. thymol

POTENTIAL SUBSTITUTIONS: Other Fir species, Scots Pine

THERAPEUTIC APPLICATIONS

INDICATIONS	METHOD OF APPLICATION	PAIRS WELL WITH
Respiratory System: Respiratory infections, bronchitis, difficulty breathing, sinusitis, spasmodic coughs	Personal inhaler, diffuser, nebulizing diffuser, chest salve, steam inhalation	Blue Gum Eucalyptus, Frankincense, Juniper Berry, Lemon, Niaouli, Peppermint, Scots Pine, Rosemary ct. cineole or Rosemary ct. camphor, Hemlock Spruce, Tea Tree, Thyme ct. linalool or Thyme ct. thymol
Psyche/emotions: Mental or emotional fatigue, anxiety. Uplifting, cleansing, clarifying. Relieves stress (by encouraging deep expansive breathing)	Personal inhaler, aromatic baths, salt scrub, body oil	Bergamot, Black Pepper, Blue Gum Eucalyptus, Frankincense, Juniper Berry, Lavender, Lemon, Peppermint, Scots Pine, Rosemary ct. cineole, Hemlock Spruce

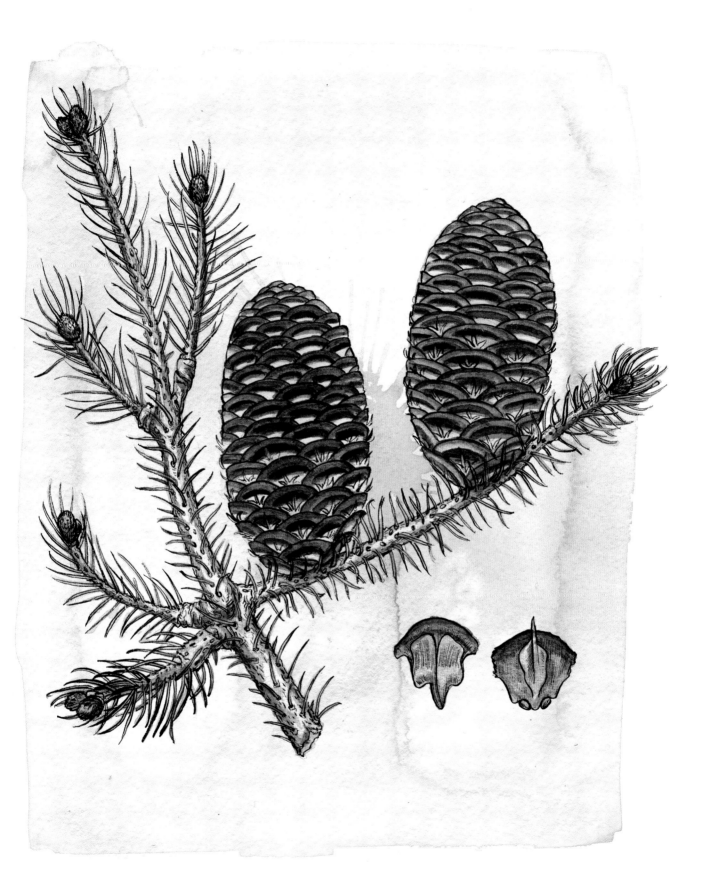

GOLDENROD

Goldenrod (*Solidago canadensis*, Asteraceae) essential oil is steam distilled using the vibrant yellow goldenrod flowers. Often confused with ragweed, goldenrod plant is rarely the cause of allergies. Indeed, the essential oil may actually provide some relief. Offering a vibrant, inspiring yet balanced earthy approach, goldenrod appears to have a balancing action on the autonomic nervous system. In other words, it is beneficial during times of stress or when one is feeling overwhelmed with too much on the plate, so to speak. This essential oil also pairs well with many of the conifer essential oils, such as hemlock spruce, Scots pine, and pinyon pine, to offer a meadow and forest-like aroma that also calms and encourages a deepening and expansion of the breath.

SOURCE COUNTRIES: Canada, United States

CORE COMPONENTS: Sesquiterpenes (germacrene D), esters (bornyl acetate), monoterpenes (d-limonene, α-pinene, β-pinene, sabinene, myrcene)

SAFETY: No known contraindications or cautions

CONSERVATION: Not yet assessed

BLENDING WITH GOLDENROD

AROMA: Green, slightly bitter yet sweet, mildly musty

SYSTEM AFFINITY: Respiratory

BLENDS WELL WITH: Bergamot Mint, Cardamom, Carrot Seed, Roman Chamomile, Clary Sage, Copaiba, Coriander Seed, Cypress, Helichrysum, Inula, Lemon, Melissa, Niaouli, Pinyon Pine, Scots Pine, Hemlock Spruce, Tea Tree, Vetiver, Yarrow

POTENTIAL SUBSTITUTIONS: Scots Pine, Pinyon Pine, Tea Tree

THERAPEUTIC APPLICATIONS

INDICATIONS	METHOD OF APPLICATION	PAIRS WELL WITH
Respiratory system: Catarrh, astringent (drippy mucus), allergies	Steam inhalation, personal inhaler, chest salve	Cardamom, Cypress, Lemon, Niaouli, Pinyon Pine, Scots Pine, Hemlock Spruce, Tea Tree, Yarrow
Psyche/emotions: Stress, anxiety, feelings of being overwhelmed or over stimulated, irritability, undernourishment	Personal inhaler, diffuser, roll-on, diffuser	Bergamot Mint, Cardamom, Roman Chamomile, Clary Sage, Copaiba, Coriander Seed, Cypress, Lemon, Melissa, Pinyon Pine, Scots Pine, Hemlock Spruce, Vetiver, Yarrow

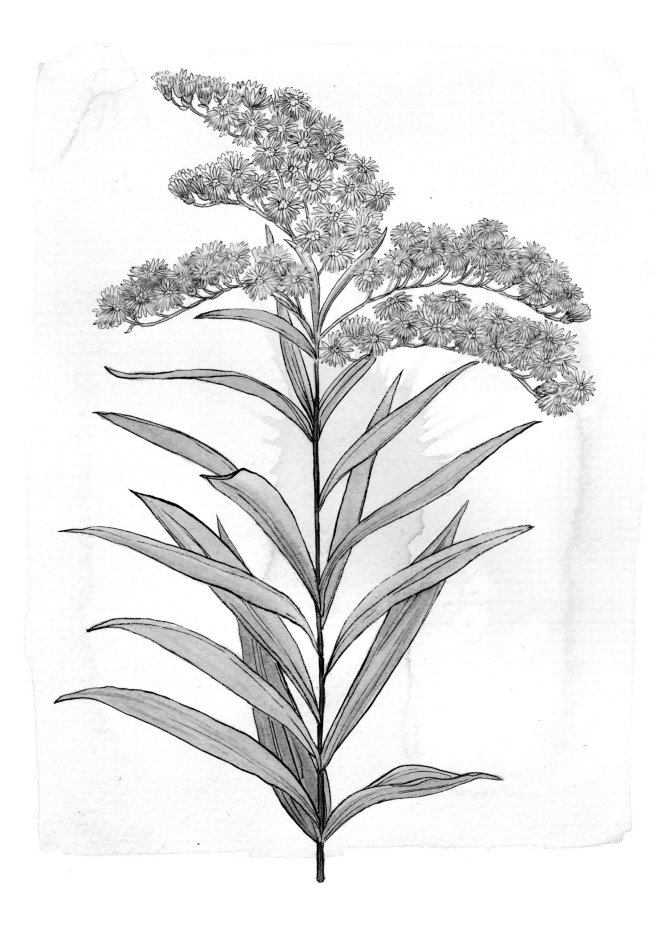

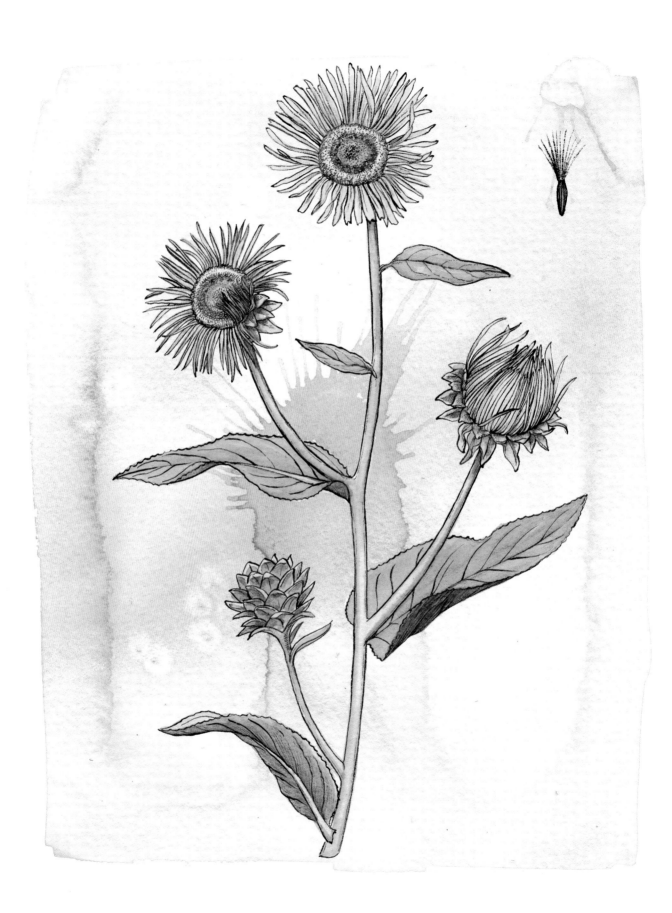

INULA

Native to the Mediterranean, **Inula** (*Dittrichia graveolens syn. Inula graveolens*, Asteraceae) essential oil is steam distilled using the flowers and flowering tops of inula. This essential oil has a beautiful rich emerald green color. What makes the oil green? When the plant material is distilled in a copper still, some trace components in this oil form complexes with copper, and voila, the essential oils turns out emerald green. When it is distilled in stainless steel, the oil is yellowish clear.[12]

SOURCE COUNTRY: Corsica (French Island)

CORE COMPONENTS: Bornyl acetate, borneol, γ-cadinene, camphene, T-cadinol

SAFETY: No known cautions or contraindications

CONSERVATION: Not defined

BLENDING WITH INULA

AROMA: Fresh, clean, light

SYSTEM AFFINITIES: Respiratory

BLENDS WELL WITH: Blue Gum Eucalyptus, Laurel, Lemon, Green Myrtle, Niaouli

POTENTIAL SUBSTITUTIONS: Blue Gum Eucalyptus, Green Myrtle

THERAPEUTIC APPLICATIONS

INDICATIONS	METHOD OF APPLICATION	PAIRS WELL WITH
Respiratory system: Sinus infections, bronchitis, lung congestion, upper respiratory congestion, spasmodic coughs, lethargy, asthma, sinus congestion	Steam inhalations, nebulizing diffuser, personal inhaler	Blue Gum Eucalyptus, Laurel, Lemon, Green Myrtle, Niaouli

SWEET MARJORAM

Native to Turkey and naturalized throughout the Mediterranean area, **Sweet Marjoram** (*Origanum majorana*, Lamiaceae) essential oil is steam distilled using the flowering tops of the marjoram plant. Sweet marjoram can help us to accept any deep loss, especially when combined with oils of cypress and rose.

SOURCE COUNTRIES: France, Germany, and Egypt

CORE CHEMICAL COMPONENTS: Terpinen-4-ol, cis-sabinene hydrate, linalyl acetate

SAFETY: No known contraindications or cautions

CONSERVATION: Not defined

BLENDING WITH SWEET MARJORAM

AROMA: Spicy, herbaceous

SYSTEM AFFINITIES: Respiratory, musculoskeletal

BLENDS WELL WITH: Angelica Root, Basil ct. linalool, Bergamot, German Chamomile, Roman Chamomile, Clary Sage, Copaiba, Cypress, Sweet Fennel, Geranium, Juniper Berry, Katafray, Lavender, Lemongrass, Mandarin, Melissa, Green Myrtle, Peppermint, Plai, Rose, Rosemary ct. verbenone, Blue Tansy

POTENTIAL SUBSTITUTIONS: Clary Sage, Lavender, Roman Chamomile, Ginger

THERAPEUTIC APPLICATIONS

INDICATIONS	METHOD OF APPLICATION	PAIRS WELL WITH
Respiratory system: Spasmodic coughs, bronchitis, sinusitis, flu, allergies, hay fever, colds	Steam inhalation, chest salve, personal inhaler, diffuser	Cypress, Juniper Berry, Katafray, Lavender, Green Myrtle, Peppermint, Plai, Rosemary ct. verbenone
Musculoskeletal system: Muscular or joint aches and pains, rheumatic aches and pains, joint swelling, muscle spasms, growing pain (adolescents), cramps, sciatica, carpal tunnel syndrome	Body oil, salve, gel, personal inhaler (to soothe stress)	Basil ct. linalool, Roman Chamomile, Juniper Berry, Katafray, Lavender, Lemongrass, Peppermint, Plai
Reproductive system: Dysmenorrhea, menstrual cramps	Abdominal oil, personal inhaler, roll-on	Basil ct. linalool, German Chamomile, Roman Chamomile, Clary Sage, Sweet Fennel, Geranium, Lavender, Plai, Rose
Psyche/emotions: Anxiety, insomnia, lethargy, nervous exhaustion, stress, agitation/irritability, obsessive thinking, grief	Personal inhaler, aromatic baths, diffuser, nebulizing diffuser	Angelica Root, Bergamot, German Chamomile, Roman Chamomile, Clary Sage, Geranium, Katafray, Lavender, Mandarin, Melissa, Rose

SCOTS PINE

Scots Pine (*Pinus sylvestris,* Pinaceae) essential oil is steam distilled using pine needles. Reminiscent of a relaxing and reinvigorating walk in an evergreen forest, Scots Pine has been used for its ability to support recovery from "adrenal exhaustion" or long periods of over-working. Scots pine is also a drying and decongestant essential oil, effectively removing or reducing excess of mucus in the respiratory system. Its gentleness supports strength and resiliency during recovery from illness.

SOURCE COUNTRY: France

CORE COMPONENTS: α-pinene, delta-3-carene

SAFETY: Due to the monoterpene content, it is important that the essential oil be stored properly (in a dark container in the refrigerator or in a cold room away from sunlight and heat). Oxidized essential oils should not be used in body care products or formulations designed for dermal application. The essential oil can, however, be used for cleaning products.

CONSERVATION: Not yet assessed

BLENDING WITH SCOTS PINE

AROMA: Balsamic, woody, piney

SYSTEM AFFINITIES: Respiratory, musculoskeletal

BLENDS WELL WITH: Black Pepper, Cypress, Inula, Juniper Berry, Lavender, Lemon, Sweet Marjoram, Niaouli, Petitgrain, Hemlock Spruce, Valerian, Ylang Ylang

POTENTIAL SUBSTITUTIONS: Maritime Pine, Black Spruce

THERAPEUTIC APPLICATIONS

INDICATIONS	METHOD OF APPLICATION	PAIRS WELL WITH
Respiratory system: Shallow breathing, bronchitis, catarrh, moist coughs, sinusitis, sore throat, allergies, respiratory infections, sinus or general respiratory congestion	Personal inhaler, chest oil, chest salve	Cypress, Inula, Sweet Marjoram, Niaouli, Hemlock Spruce
Musculoskeletal system: Muscular aches and pains, arthritis, rheumatism, neuralgia, joint pain, sciatica, muscle cramps	Body oil, unscented lotion, gel	Black Pepper, Juniper Berry, Lavender, Lemon, Sweet Marjoram
Psyche/emotions: Nervous exhaustion, fatigue, depression, mental fatigue adrenal depletion/fatigue, nervous asthenia	Personal inhaler, roll-on	Lavender, Lemon, Sweet Marjoram, Petitgrain, Hemlock Spruce, Valerian, Ylang Ylang

GREEN MYRTLE

Green Myrtle (*Myrtus communis*, Myrtaceae) essential oil is steam distilled using the leaves from the small evergreen shrub. Green myrtle inspires deep and expansive breathing, supports elimination of mucus congestion, and supports the immune system in fighting common respiratory ailments such as the cold or flu.

SOURCE COUNTRY: France

CORE COMPONENTS: α-pinene, 1,8 cineole, limonene, myrtenyl acetate, linalool

SAFETY: No known contraindications or cautions

CONSERVATION: Least concern

BLENDING WITH GREEN MYRTLE

AROMA: Camphoraceous, warm, somewhat sweet, fresh

SYSTEM AFFINITIES: Respiratory

BLENDS WELL WITH: Frankincense, Blue Gum Eucalyptus, Laurel, Niaouli, Rosemary ct. cineole or Rosemary ct. camphor, Saro, Thyme ct. linalool or Thyme ct. thymol

POTENTIAL SUBSTITUTIONS: Blue Gum Eucalyptus, Laurel, Rosemary ct. cineole, Saro

THERAPEUTIC APPLICATIONS

INDICATIONS	METHOD OF APPLICATION	PAIRS WELL WITH
Respiratory system: Mucus congestion, bronchitis, excess catarrh, flu, common cold, asthma, chronic smoker's cough, sinusitis, respiratory infections, lung congestion	Steam inhalation, personal inhaler, nebulizing diffuser, chest salve	Frankincense, Blue Gum Eucalyptus, Laurel, Niaouli, Rosemary ct. cineole, Saro, Thyme ct. thymol
Musculoskeletal system: Muscular aches and pains, joint stiffness or pain	Body oil, salve, unscented cream or lotion	Frankincense, Blue Gum Eucalyptus, Laurel, Niaouli, Rosemary ct. cineole or Rosemary ct. camphor

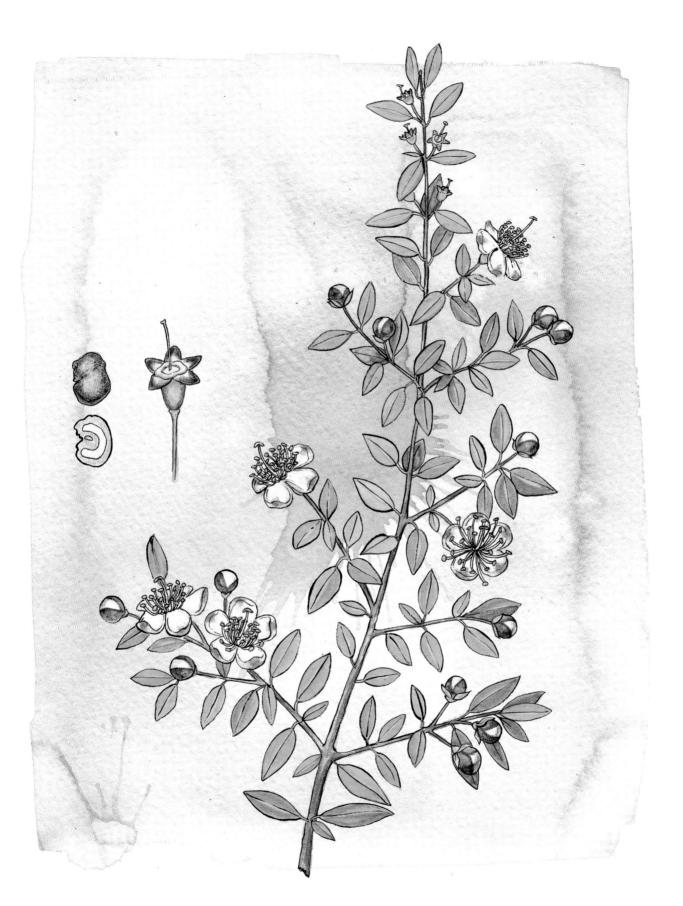

NIAOULI

Niaouli (*Melaleuca quinquenervia*, Myrtaceae) essential oil is steam distilled using the leaves of the niaouli tree. Popularized by esteemed aromatherapy educator and author Dr. Kurt Schnaubelt, niaouli shines in its ability to support and enhance immunity and the body's ability to deal with infection.

SOURCE COUNTRIES: Australia, Madagascar, and New Caledonia

CORE COMPONENTS: 1,8 cineole

CAUTION FOR CHILDREN: Essential oils high in 1,8 cineole can cause central nervous system and breathing problems in young children. Do not apply to or near the face of infants or children.

CONSERVATION: Not defined

BLENDING WITH NIAOULI

AROMA: Camphoraceous, eucalyptus-like with pungent note

SYSTEM AFFINITIES: Respiratory, immune, skin

BLENDS WELL WITH: Cistus, Cypress, Eucalyptus, Lemon, Green Myrtle, Petitgrain, Rosemary (all chemotypes), Saro, Blue Tansy, Tea Tree, Thyme ct. thymol

POTENTIAL SUBSTITUTIONS: Saro, Tea Tree, Laurel

THERAPEUTIC APPLICATIONS

INDICATIONS	METHOD OF APPLICATION	PAIRS WELL WITH
Respiratory system: Respiratory infections: bronchitis, colds, sinusitis, chest infections, bacterial or viral catarrhal colds, pharyngitis	Steam inhalation, personal inhaler, chest salve or oil	Cypress, Eucalyptus, Lemon, Green Myrtle, Rosemary ct. cineole, Saro, Tea Tree, Thyme ct. thymol
Skin: Acne, athlete's foot, fungal infections, wounds, psoriasis, acne, sores, fissures, boils, scar tissue, ulcers, fungal or parasitic skin infections. Protects from burns from radiation	Gel, cleanser	Cistus, Cypress, Lemon, Petitgrain, Rosemary ct. verbenone, Blue Tansy, Tea Tree

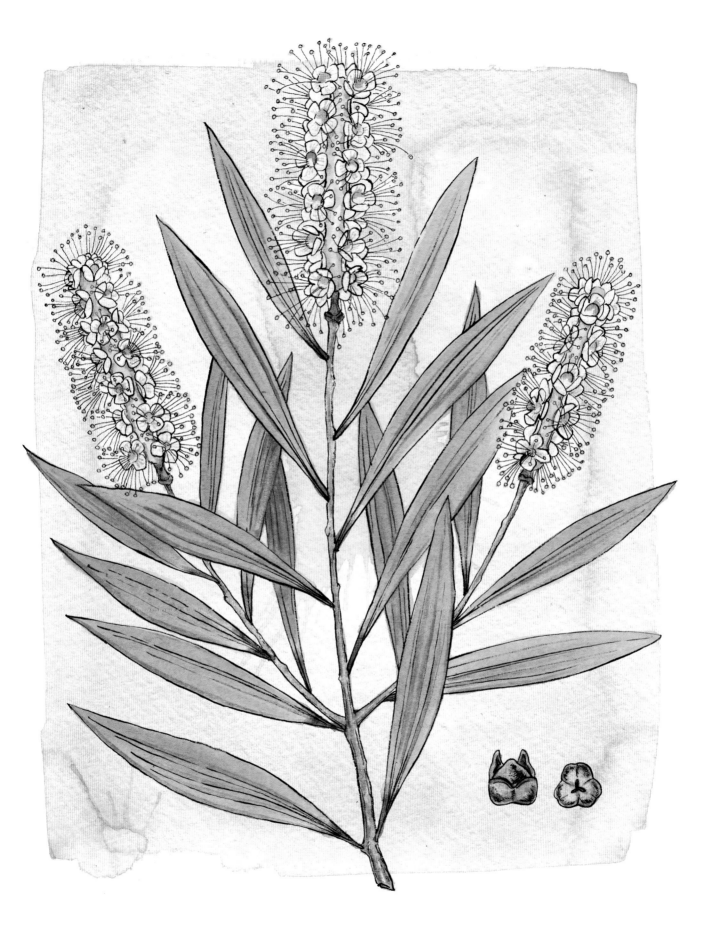

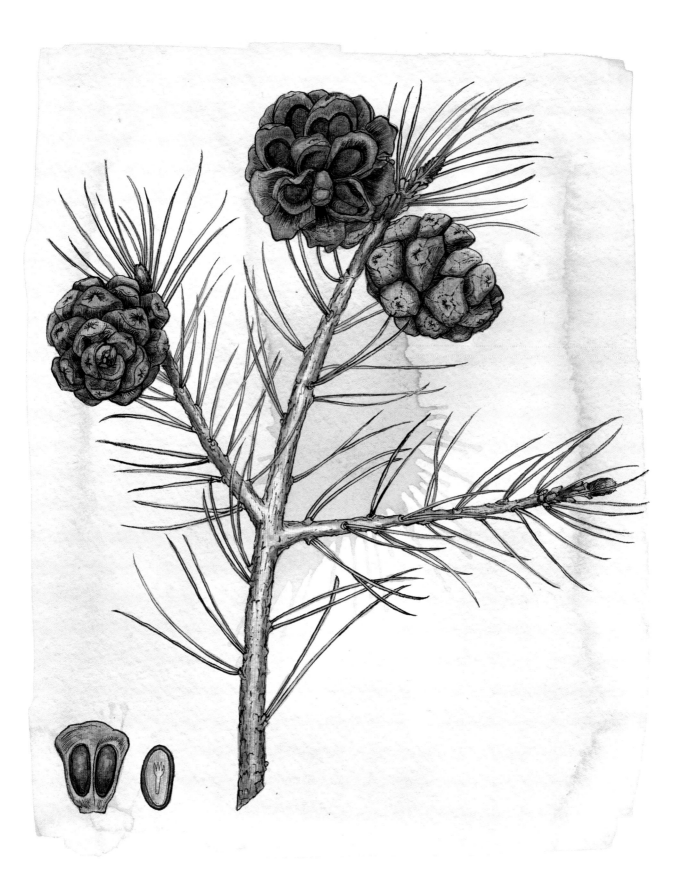

PINYON PINE

Native to southwestern North America, **Pinyon Pine** (*Pinus edulis*, Pinaceae) essential oil is steam distilled using needles, twigs, and branches of this fragrant tree. The resin from the tree can be infused into jojoba oil to make an incredibly aromatic oil that not only relieves muscular aches and pains and respiratory congestion, but also uplifts and inspires!

SOURCE COUNTRY: Southwest United States

CORE COMPONENTS: α-pinene, β-pinene, β-phellandrene

DERMAL CAUTION: Due to monoterpene content, potential skin sensitization if the essential oil oxidizes. Avoid old or oxidized essential oils.

CONSERVATION: Not yet assessed

BLENDING WITH PINYON PINE

AROMA: Soft floral-fruity, balsamic, resin-like, earthy

SYSTEM AFFINITIES: Respiratory

BLENDS WELL WITH: Angelica Root, Basil ct. linalool, Himalayan Cedarwood, Cistus, Copaiba, Cypress, Balsam Fir, Frankincense, Goldenrod, Grapefruit, Lemon, Patchouli, Hemlock Spruce, Saro, Valerian

POTENTIAL SUBSTITUTIONS: Balsam Fir, Himalayan Cedarwood, Hemlock Spruce

THERAPEUTIC APPLICATIONS

INDICATIONS	METHOD OF APPLICATION	PAIRS WELL WITH:
Respiratory system: Asthma, bronchitis, catarrh, coughs, sinusitis, sore throat, allergies. Expands breathing	Personal inhaler, steam inhalation, chest salve	Cypress, Balsam Fir, Frankincense, Goldenrod, Lemon, Hemlock Spruce, Saro
Musculoskeletal system: Muscular aches and pains, arthritis, rheumatism, joint pain	Gel, lotion, body oil, salve	Basil ct. linalool, Himalayan Cedarwood, Grapefruit, Lemon, Hemlock Spruce
Psyche/emotions: Nervous exhaustion, fatigue, depression, mental fatigue	Personal inhaler, diffuser, roll-on	Angelica Root, Basil ct. linalool, Himalayan Cedarwood, Frankincense, Grapefruit, Lemon, Patchouli, Hemlock Spruce, Saro, Valerian

ROSEMARY

Rosemary (*Rosmarinus officinalis*, Lamiaceae) produces three well-known chemotypes: ct. cineole, ct. camphor, and ct. verbenone. Each chemotype of Rosemary has a slightly different aroma and affinity although often they are used interchangeably with one another. The ct. verbenone tends to be the most expensive and is used in regenerative skin care. There are three well-known chemotypes for Rosemary:

ROSEMARY CT. CINEOLE

SOURCE COUNTRIES: Morocco, France, Spain, South Africa, and Tunisia

CORE COMPONENT: 1,8 cineole, α-pinene, camphor, and β-caryophyllene

SAFETY: Avoid application of 1,8 cineole–rich essential oils to the face or near the nose of infants and children under the age of 5 years. Do not instill 1,8 cineole-rich essential oils into the nose of infants or children. Use low dilutions (less than 1 percent) with children aged 3 to 7 years.

CONSERVATION: Least concerned

BLENDING WITH ROSEMARY CT. CINEOLE

AROMA: Eucalyptus-like

SYSTEM AFFINITIES: Respiratory

BLENDS WELL WITH: Cardamom, Cypress, Juniper Berry, Laurel, Lavender, Lemon, Green Myrtle, Plai

POTENTIAL SUBSTITUTIONS: Blue Gum Eucalyptus, Laurel

THERAPEUTIC APPLICATIONS

INDICATIONS	METHOD OF APPLICATION	PAIRS WELL WITH
Respiratory system: Sinusitis, mucus, bronchitis, congestion	Steam inhalation, personal inhaler, chest salve, chest oil, aromatic baths	Cardamom, Cinnamon Leaf, Blue Gum Eucalyptus, Laurel
Musculoskeletal system: Muscular aches and pains, stiffness, fatigue	Gel, unscented lotion, body oil, salve	Bergamot Mint, Juniper Berry, Lavender, Lemongrass, Peppermint
Psyche/emotions: Poor memory, fatigue, foggy thinking, inability to concentrate. Clears the mind	Personal inhaler, diffusion, nebulizing diffusion, roll-on, salt scrub	Cardamom, Blue Gum Eucalyptus, Laurel, Lemon, Peppermint

ROSEMARY CT. CAMPHOR

SOURCE COUNTRIES: Spain, Croatia, and S. Africa

CORE COMPONENT: camphor, 1,8 cineole, α-pinene

SAFETY: Avoid application of 1,8 cineole–rich essential oils to the face or near the nose of infants and children under the age of 5 years. Do not instill 1,8 cineole-rich essential oils into the nose of infants or children. Use low dilutions (less than 1 percent) with children aged 3 to 7 years.

CONSERVATION: Least concerned

BLENDING WITH ROSEMARY CT. CAMPHOR

AROMA: Camphoraceous, eucalyptus-like

SYSTEM AFFINITY: Musculoskeletal

BLENDS WELL WITH: Cardamom, Cypress, Juniper Berry, Laurel, Lavender, Lemon, Green Myrtle, Plai, Peppermint, Scots Pine, Rosemary ct. cineole, Hemlock Spruce, Thyme ct. thymol or Thyme ct. linalool

POTENTIAL SUBSTITUTIONS: Rosemary ct. cineole, Laurel

THERAPEUTIC APPLICATIONS

INDICATIONS	METHOD OF APPLICATION	PAIRS WELL WITH
Musculoskeletal system: Muscular aches, cramps, spasms, neuralgic rheumatic pain, arthritic conditions	Body oil, salve, gel, unscented cream or lotion	Bergamot Mint, Clary Sage, Juniper Berry, Laurel, Lavender, Peppermint, Plai, Vetiver
Psyche/emotions: Low energy, depression, fatigue, malaise, poor memory, inability to concentrate	Personal inhaler, roll-on	Juniper Berry, Laurel, Peppermint. Rosemary ct. cineole

ROSEMARY CT. VERBENONE

SOURCE COUNTRIES: France, Corsica

CORE COMPONENT: α-pinene, 1,8 cineole, camphor, verbenone

SAFETY: Avoid application of 1,8 cineole–rich essential oils to the face or near the nose of infants and children under the age of 5 years. Do not instill 1,8 cineole-rich essential oils into the nose of infants or children. Use low dilutions (less than 1percent) with children aged 3 to 7 years.

CONSERVATION: Least concerned

BLENDING WITH ROSEMARY CT. VERBENONE

AROMA: Slightly earthy eucalyptus-like

SYSTEM AFFINITY: Respiratory

BLENDS WELL WITH: Carrot Seed, Cypress, Helichrysum, Juniper Berry, Laurel, Lavender, Lemon, Plai, Rosemary ct. cineole, Hemlock Spruce, Thyme ct. thymol or Thyme ct. linalool

POTENTIAL SUBSTITUTIONS: Helichrysum, Carrot Seed

THERAPEUTIC APPLICATIONS

INDICATIONS	METHOD OF APPLICATION	PAIRS WELL WITH
Skin: Rosacea, acne, seborrhea (oily skin with congestion), varicose veins, wounds. Promotes microcirculation, skin care	Facial or body cleanser, unscented cream or lotion, gel, facial or body oil, salve	Calendula CO2, Carrot Seed, German Chamomile, Helichrysum, Lavender, Petitgrain, Thyme ct. linalool, Yarrow
Psyche/emotions: Restores psychological balance, clears mind	Personal inhaler, diffusion, roll-on	Rosemary ct. cineole

RAVINTSARA CT. CINEOLE

Ravintsara ct. cineole (*Cinnamomum camphora*, Lauraceae) essential oil is steam distilled using the leaves of the tree.

SOURCE COUNTRY: Madagascar

CORE COMPONENTS: 1,8 cineole, sabinene, α-pinene, β-pinene, α-terpineol

CAUTION FOR CHILDREN: Avoid application of 1,8 cineole-rich essential oils to the face or near the nose of infants and children under the age of 3 years. Do not instill 1,8 cineole-rich essential oils into the nose of infants or children under the age of 7 years.

CONSERVATION: Not defined

BLENDING WITH RAVINTSARA CT. CINEOLE

AROMA: Pungent, spicy, warming, slightly woody, light

SYSTEM AFFINITIES: Respiratory, musculoskeletal

BLENDS WELL WITH: Cypress, Eucalyptus, Green Myrtle, Niaouli, Sandalwood

POTENTIAL SUBSTITUTIONS: Eucalyptus globulus, Niaouli, Green Myrtle

THERAPEUTIC APPLICATIONS

INDICATIONS	METHOD OF APPLICATION	PAIRS WELL WITH:
Respiratory system: bronchitis, catarrh, upper or lower respiratory tract infection, influenza, sinusitis, allergies	Steam inhalation, personal inhaler, chest salve, chest oil, nebulizing diffuser	Cypress, Eucalyptus globulus, Green Myrtle, Niaouli, Sandalwood
Musculoskeletal system: muscular aches and pains, arthritis, muscular pain caused by excess coughing	Body oil, gel, salve, aromatic baths	Cypress, Eucalyptus globulus, Green Myrtle

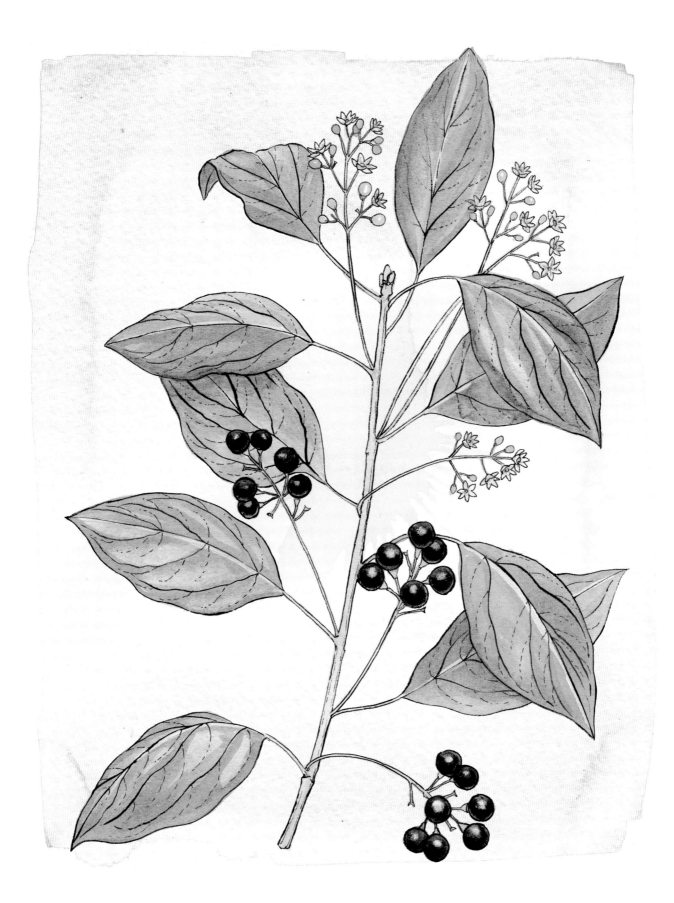

SARO

Saro (*Cinnamosma fragrans*, Canellaceae) essential oil is steam distilled using the leaves of the saro tree. Saro gained its notoriety for its exception benefits for the respiratory system. Diffusing saro into your space during the autumn and winter months could help prevent common seasonal illnesses.

SOURCE COUNTRY: Madagascar

CORE COMPONENTS: 1,8 cineole, α-pinene, β-pinene, linalool, terpinen-4-ol

CAUTION FOR CHILDREN: Avoid application of 1,8 cineole-rich essential oils to the face or near the nose of infants and children under the age of 5 years. Do not instill 1,8 cineole-rich essential oils into the nose of infants or children. Use low dilutions (less than 1 percent) with children between 3 and 7 years.

CONSERVATION: Not yet assessed

BLENDING WITH SARO

AROMA: Eucalyptus-like, fresh, clean, green, warm

SYSTEM AFFINITIES: Respiratory

BLENDS WELL WITH: Cypress, Blue Gum Eucalyptus, Balsam Fir, Lavender, Lemon, Green Myrtle, Peppermint, Hemlock Spruce, Thyme ct. thymol or Thyme ct. linalool

POTENTIAL SUBSTITUTIONS: Blue Gum Eucalyptus, Laurel, Rosemary ct. cineole

THERAPEUTIC APPLICATIONS

INDICATIONS	METHOD OF APPLICATION	PAIRS WELL WITH
Respiratory system: Acute or chronic bronchitis, moist or dry coughs, the common cold, sinusitis, dry cough. Protective and preventative to common winter ailments	Personal inhaler, diffuser, nebulizing diffuser, steam inhalation	Cypress, Blue Gum Eucalyptus, Balsam Fir, Lavender, Lemon, Green Myrtle, Peppermint, Hemlock Spruce, Tea Tree, Thyme ct. thymol or Thyme ct. linalool
Psyche/emotions: Foggy or cluttered thinking, lack of energy, lethargy	Personal inhaler, roll-on, salt scrub	Cypress, Balsam Fir, Lavender, Lemon, Green Myrtle, Hemlock Spruce

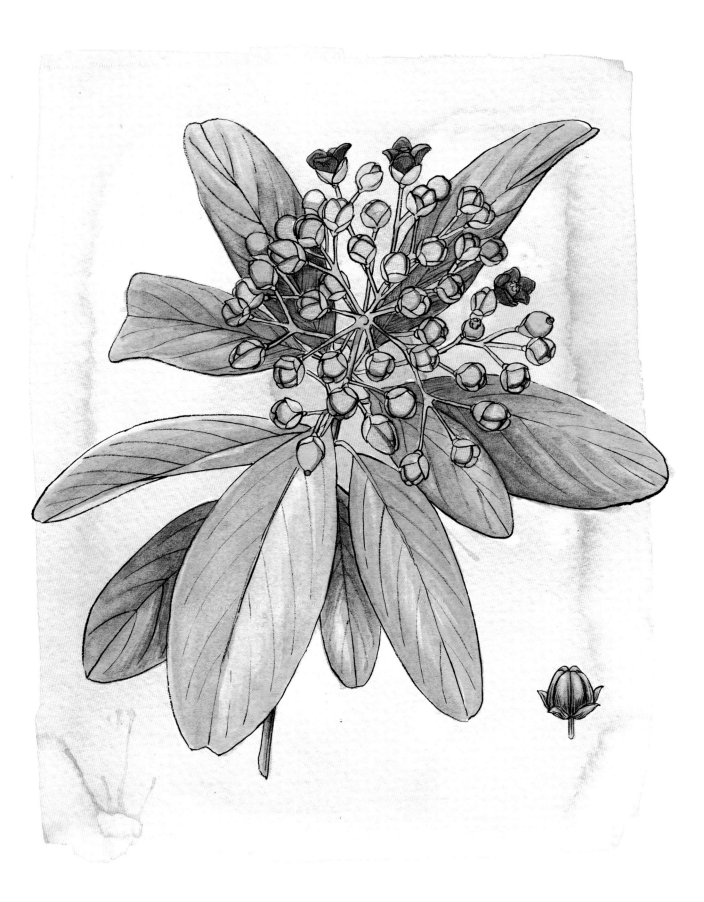

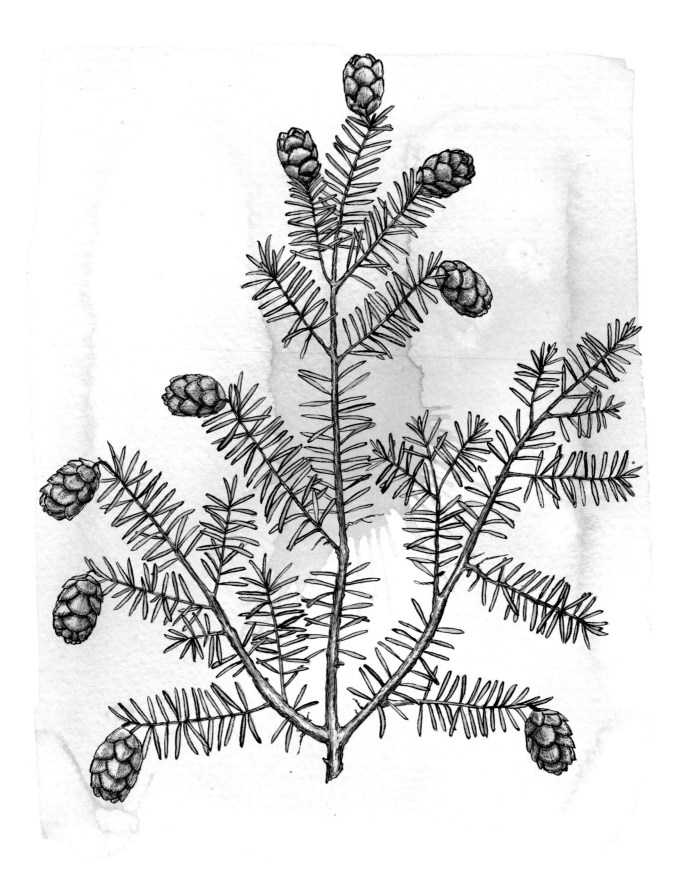

HEMLOCK SPRUCE

Hemlock Spruce (*Tsuga canadensis*, Pinaceae) essential oil is steam distilled using hemlock needles. Like Scots pine, hemlock spruce is beneficial when one is feeling burned out and in need of the forest, so to speak. Hemlock inspires deep, expansive breathing while supporting the health of the respiratory system.

SOURCE COUNTRY: Canada

CORE COMPONENTS: Bornyl acetate, camphene

DERMAL CAUTION: Potential skin sensitizer if the oil is oxidized. Avoid older oils and store correctly.

CONSERVATION: Least concern

BLENDING WITH HEMLOCK SPRUCE

AROMA: Pungent, spicy, warming, slightly woody, light

SYSTEM AFFINITIES: Respiratory, musculoskeletal

BLENDS WELL WITH: Balsam Fir, Bergamot, Bergamot Mint, Cistus, Cypress, Fingerroot, Frankincense, Scots Pine, Goldenrod, Grapefruit, Lemon, Lemongrass, Green Myrtle, Neroli, Scots Pine, Pinyon Pine, Rosemary ct. cineole, Saro, Blue Tansy

POTENTIAL SUBSTITUTIONS: Balsam Fir, Scots Pine, Pinyon Pine

THERAPEUTIC APPLICATIONS

INDICATIONS	METHOD OF APPLICATION	PAIRS WELL WITH
Respiratory system: Colds, flu, bronchitis, catarrh	Steam inhalation, personal inhaler, chest salve, diffuser, nebulizing diffuser	Balsam Fir, Cypress, Frankincense, Scots Pine, Goldenrod, Lemon, Green Myrtle, Scots Pine, Pinyon Pine, Saro
Musculoskeletal system: Muscular aches and pains, muscle or joint stiffness, rheumatic pain, tension	Gel, lotion, body oil	Bergamot Mint, Grapefruit, Lemon, Lemongrass, Scots Pine, Pinyon Pine
Psyche/emotions: Both general and profound fatigue, mental and emotional exhaustion, anxiety, stress. Gives stamina when one is tired	Personal inhaler, roll-on, body butter, salt scrub	Balsam Fir, Bergamot, Bergamot Mint, Cistus, Cypress, Fingerroot, Frankincense, Scots Pine, Goldenrod, Grapefruit, Lemon, Lemongrass, Green Myrtle, Neroli, Scots Pine, Pinyon Pine, Rosemary ct. cineole, Saro, Blue Tansy

BLUE TANSY

Blue Tansy, also known as Moroccan chamomile (*Tanacetum annuum*, Asteraceae), essential oil is steam distilled using the flowering tops. Blue tansy gained its popularity as an anti-inflammatory, anti-histaminic, and anti-allergenic essential oil used to ease allergy symptoms in the springtime.

SOURCE COUNTRY: Morocco

CORE COMPONENTS: Sabinene, β-pinene, myrcene, α-phellandrene, p-cymene, chamazulene, camphor

SAFETY: No known concerns or contraindications

CONSERVATION: Not defined

BLENDING WITH BLUE TANSY

AROMA: Rich, herbaceous, apple-like sweetness

SYSTEM AFFINITIES: Skin, respiratory

BLENDS WELL WITH: German Chamomile, Coriander Seed, Lavender, Niaouli, Peppermint, Hemlock Spruce

POTENTIAL SUBSTITUTIONS: German Chamomile

THERAPEUTIC APPLICATIONS

INDICATIONS	METHOD OF APPLICATION	PAIRS WELL WITH
Respiratory system: Seasonal allergies, hay fever, asthma, emphysema	Personal inhaler, chest salve	German Chamomile, Coriander Seed, Lavender, Niaouli, Peppermint, Hemlock Spruce
Skin: Inflamed skin conditions, itching, itching caused by allergy, eczema, dry irritated skin	Unscented cream or lotion, facial oil, body oil	German Chamomile, Lavender, Niaouli
Psyche/emotions: Irritability, easily overheating, anger, frustration	Personal inhaler, roll-on	German Chamomile, Coriander Seed, Lavender, Hemlock Spruce

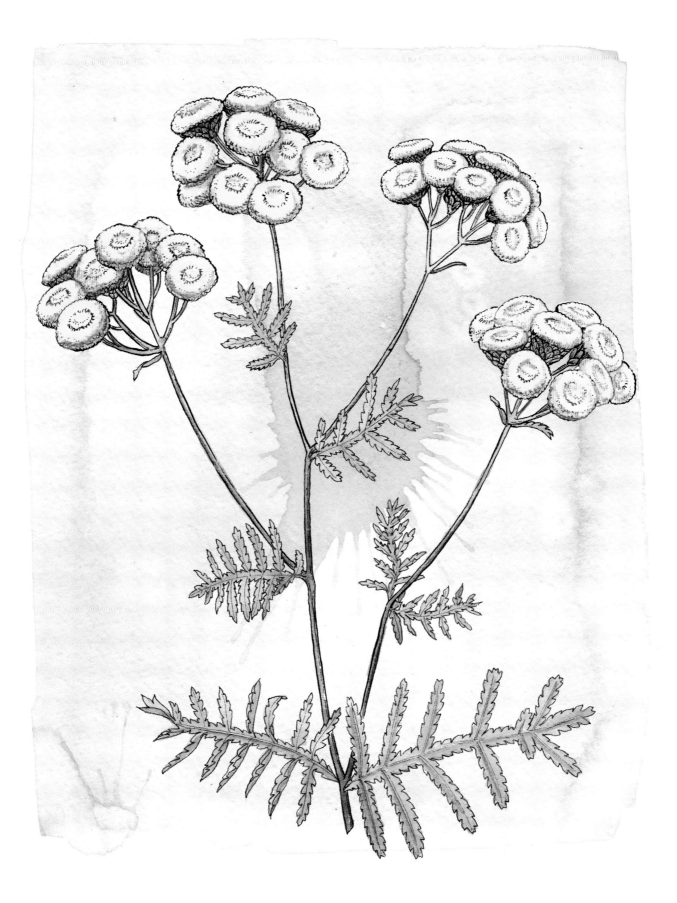

CAPE CHAMOMILE

Cape Chamomile (*Eriocephalus punctulatus*, Asteraceae) essential oil is steam distilled using the leaves of the cape chamomile shrub. As a member of the chamomile tribe, cape chamomile soothes inflammation, relaxes muscle tension, and relieves anxiety. It has a light blue color due to the presence of a small amount of chamazulene, a component that contributes to its ability to reduce inflammation.

SOURCE COUNTRY: South Africa

CORE COMPONENTS: Rich in esters including 2-methylbutyl 2-methylpropanoate and linalyl acetate

SAFETY: No known contraindications

CONSERVATION: Not defined

BLENDING WITH CAPE CHAMOMILE

AROMA: Sweet, fruity, apple-like, strong

SYSTEM AFFINITIES: Skin

BLENDS WELL WITH: Calendula CO2, Himalayan Cedarwood, German Chamomile, Roman Chamomile, Copaiba, Coriander Seed, Fingerroot, Grapefruit, Katafray, Lavender, Lemon, Mandarin, Myrrh, Neroli, Peppermint, Vetiver, Yarrow, Ylang Ylang

POTENTIAL SUBSTITUTIONS: German Chamomile, Lavender, Roman Chamomile, English Chamomile

THERAPEUTIC APPLICATIONS

INDICATIONS	METHOD OF APPLICATION	PAIRS WELL WITH
Skin: Itchy or inflamed skin conditions, insect bites, sunburn, acne, psoriasis May be used undiluted for acute skin conditions such as bug bites, chiggers, and stings, as well as for acne spots.	Cream, lotion, body oil for localized application, body butter, gel, salve, roll-on	Calendula CO2, Himalayan Cedarwood, German Chamomile, Roman Chamomile, Copaiba, Lavender, Lemon, Myrrh, Neroli, Yarrow
Psyche/emotions: Anxiety, feelings of being overwhelmed, irritability	Personal inhaler, salt inhaler, diffuser, roll-on	Himalayan Cedarwood, German Chamomile, Roman Chamomile, Copaiba, Coriander Seed, Grapefruit, Katafray, Lavender, Lemon, Mandarin, Myrrh, Neroli, Vetiver, Yarrow, Ylang Ylang

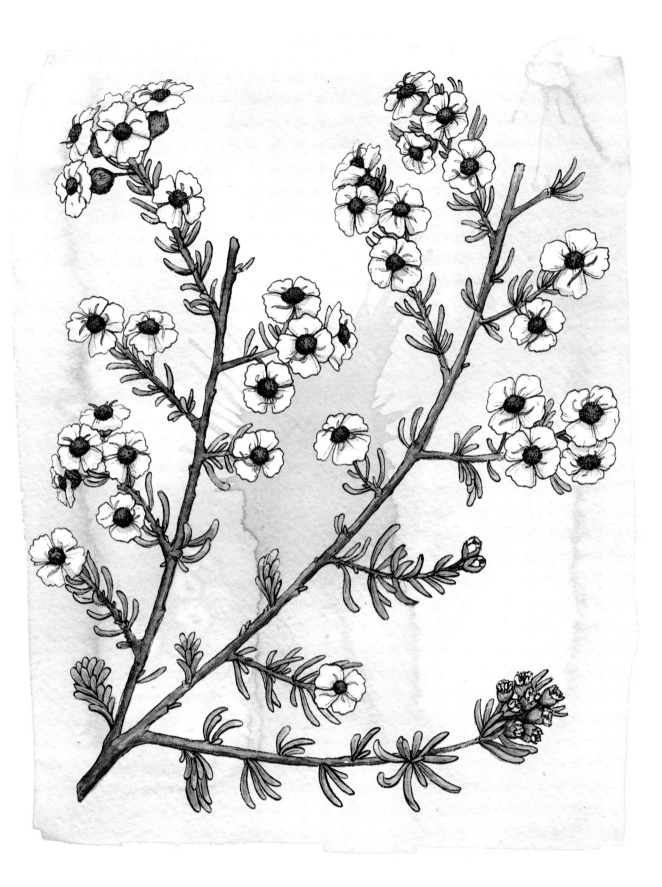

CARROT SEED

Carrot Seed (*Daucus carota* subsp. *carota*, Apiaceae) essential oil is steam distilled using dried carrot seeds. This plant species is cultivated for an essential oil rich in the sesquiterpene alcohol carotol, considered to be one of the components responsible for carrot seed's cell regenerative powers. Used almost exclusively in skin care formulations, carrot seed also has an affinity to digestion, supporting its healthy functioning.

SOURCE COUNTRIES: France, Holland, and Hungary

CORE COMPONENTS: The sesquiterpene alcohol carotol, supported by sesquiterpenes, β-caryophyllene, daucene, β-selinene, β-bisabolene, germacrene D

SAFETY: No known contraindications

CONSERVATION: Least concern

BLENDING WITH CARROT SEED

AROMA: Tenacious, fresh, warm-spicy

SYSTEM AFFINITIES: Skin, digestive

BLENDS WELL WITH: Calendula CO2, German Chamomile, Cistus, Copaiba, Coriander Seed, Sweet Fennel, Geranium, Helichrysum, Lavender, Lemongrass, Pink Pepper, Rosemary ct. verbenone, Thyme ct. linalool, Yarrow

POTENTIAL SUBSTITUTIONS: Celery Seed, Sweet Fennel, Rosemary ct. verbenone

THERAPEUTIC APPLICATIONS

INDICATIONS	METHOD OF APPLICATION	PAIRS WELL WITH
Skin: Eczema, broken capillaries, brown spots, poor circulation in skin, wounds, age spots. Preventative against wrinkles, acne, rosacea, cellulite	Facial oil, cleanser, cream, salt scrub, salves	Calendula CO2, German Chamomile, Cistus, Copaiba, Geranium, Helichrysum, Lavender, Lemongrass, Rosemary ct. verbenone, Thyme ct. linalool, Yarrow
Digestive system: Sluggish digestion	Personal inhaler, abdominal oil, diffusion	Coriander Seed, Sweet Fennel, Lemongrass, Pink Pepper
Psyche/emotions: Anxiety, lack of clarity, emotional or mental tension, inability to let go, feelings of being weighed down	Personal inhaler, diffuser, roll-on	Coriander Seed, Sweet Fennel, Geranium, Lavender, Yarrow

GERMAN CHAMOMILE

German Chamomile (*Matricaria chamomilla* (syn. *Matricaria recutita*), Asteraceae) can reduce inflammation, support cellular regeneration, and support wound healing. It is also used to calm stress-related digestive upsets and anxiety.

SOURCE COUNTRIES: Hungary, Eastern Europe, North America, and Australia

CORE COMPONENTS: Rich in oxides and the sesquiterpene alcohol (-)-α-bisabolol

DERMAL CAUTION: People with known sensitivities to other members of the Asteraceae (Compositae) family (e.g., ragweed and daisies) may want to avoid topical application of chamomile or chamomile products.[10]

CONSERVATION: Least concern

SHELF LIFE NOTE: This essential oil is known to oxidize rapidly, turning from blue to green and then to brown. Once oxidized, it should not be used.

BLENDING WITH GERMAN CHAMOMILE

AROMA: Sweet, grassy, strong, similar to hay,

SYSTEM AFFINITIES: Skin, digestive

BLENDS WELL WITH: Black Pepper, Calendula CO2,

POTENTIAL SUBSTITUTIONS: Cape Chamomile, Copaiba, Lavender, Roman Chamomile,

THERAPEUTIC APPLICATIONS

INDICATIONS	METHOD OF APPLICATION	PAIRS WELL WITH
Skin: Eczema or Rosacea. Burns. Dry itchy skin, cuts, scrapes, slow-healing wounds, broken capillaries, acne, diaper rash.	Cleanser, cream/lotion, gel, salve, facial oil, body oil	Calendula CO$_2$, Copaiba, Helichrysum, Lavender, Patchouli, Rose, Vetiver
Digestive system: Stress-related digestive upset, general digestive complaints, cramps, colic pain	Abdominal oil, personal inhaler, roller ball	Black Pepper, Roman Chamomile, Sweet Fennel, Lavender, Peppermint
Reproductive system: PMS, cracked nipples, postpartum anxiety, and painful menstruation	Salve, cream, personal inhaler, roller ball	Cape Chamomile, Roman Chamomile, Copaiba, Clary Sage, Sweet Fennel, Geranium, Mandarin,
Musculoskeletal system: Fibromyalgia, shin splints, spasms or cramps, plantar fasciitis, tendinitis, and pain or swelling in joints	Body oil, salve, lotion	Black Pepper, Roman Chamomile, Clary Sage, Lavender, Sweet Marjoram, Peppermint, Vetiver
Psyche/emotions: Nervous irritability, mild sleep disorders, tension headaches, agitation/anger, hyperactivity in children; stress-related conditions, anxiety	Personal inhaler	Black Pepper, Calendula CO2, Cape Chamomile, Roman Chamomile, Copaiba, Clary Sage, Sweet Fennel, Lavender, Sweet Marjoram, Patchouli, Peppermint

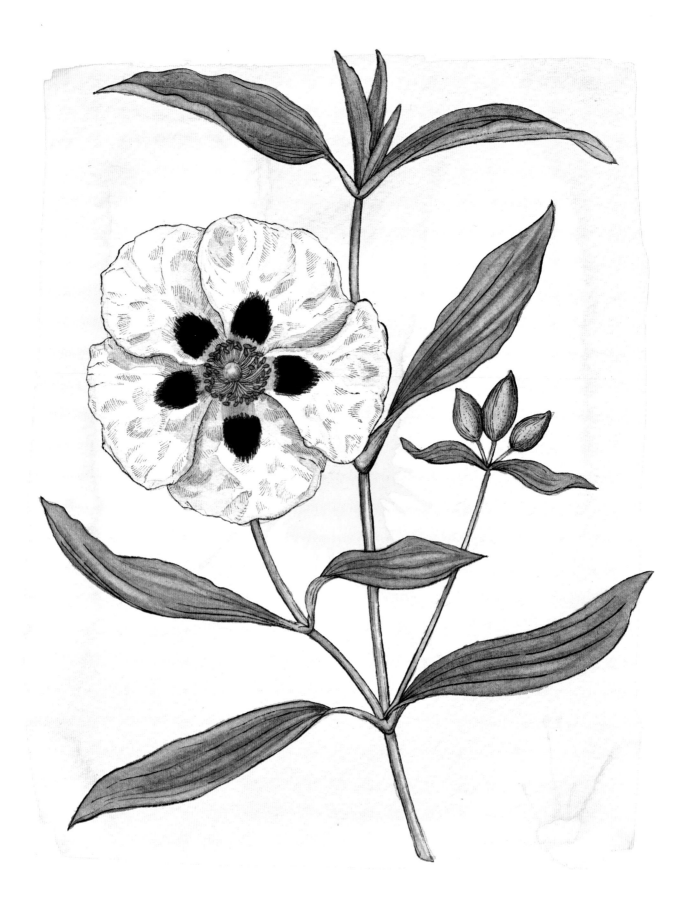

CISTUS

Cistus (*Cistus ladanifer*, Cistaceae) essential oil, also known as rockrose, is steam distilled using the dried delicate cistus flowers and leaves. Cistus essential oil is beloved for its affinity to the skin and wound healing capabilities. Cistus also displays anti-infectious and antimicrobial activity, thereby protecting the wound from infection. We recommend using it in a gel or, if possible, use Cistus hydrosol as a spray for the wound.

SOURCE COUNTRIES: Spain, Morocco, France, Portugal, and Greece (Crete)

CORE COMPONENTS: Incredibly complex chemistry with more than 250 unique components. Cistus is rich in α-pinene but is supported all around by its other components.

DERMAL CAUTION: Potential skin sensitizer if the oil is oxidized. Avoid older oils and store correctly.

CONSERVATION: Not yet assessed

BLENDING WITH CISTUS

AROMA: Warm, woody, herbaceous, crisp

SYSTEM AFFINITIES: Skin

BLENDS WELL WITH: Carrot Seed, Clary Sage, Frankincense, Helichrysum, Katafray, Lavender, Lemon, Myrrh, Neroli, Sweet Orange, Patchouli, Petitgrain, Rose, Rosemary ct. verbenone, Yarrow

POTENTIAL SUBSTITUTIONS: Yarrow, Lavender

THERAPEUTIC APPLICATIONS

INDICATIONS	METHOD OF APPLICATION	PAIRS WELL WITH
Skin: Cuts, rosacea, broken capillaries, wounds, acne, aging skin, mature skin, prematurely aging skin	Unscented cream or lotion, facial or body oil, gel	Carrot Seed, Frankincense, Helichrysum, Lavender, Lemon, Myrrh, Neroli, Patchouli, Rose, Rosemary ct. verbenone, Yarrow
Psyche/emotions: Emotional trauma, old emotional wounds	Personal inhaler, roll-on	Frankincense, Helichrysum, Katafray, Lavender, Lemon, Myrrh, Neroli, Sweet Orange, Patchouli, Petitgrain, Rose, Yarrow

COPAIBA

Copaiba (*Copaifera officinalis*, Fabaceae) essential oil is steam distilled using the resin that exudes from the cut bark of the copaiba tree. Much loved for its anti-inflammatory activity due to its high content of β-caryophyllene, copaiba is often used in body care products designed for inflamed conditions of the skin. With its gentle aroma, it also calms and soothes the nerves.

SOURCE COUNTRY: Brazil

CORE COMPONENTS: Rich in sesquiterpenes, specifically β-caryophyllene and α-copaene

SAFETY: No known contraindications or cautions

CONSERVATION: Not defined

BLENDING WITH COPAIBA

AROMA: Resinous, fresh, earthy, heavy, sweet

SYSTEM AFFINITIES: Skin, musculoskeletal

BLENDS WELL WITH: Angelica Root, Calendula CO_2, Cape Chamomile, Carrot Seed, Cistus, Cypress, Frankincense, Grapefruit, Helichrysum, Lavender, Lemon, Lemongrass, Sweet Marjoram, Sweet Orange, Petitgrain, Pinyon Pine, Thyme ct. linalool, Valerian, Yarrow, Ylang Ylang

POTENTIAL SUBSTITUTIONS: Black Pepper, Melissa, Ylang Ylang

THERAPEUTIC APPLICATIONS

INDICATIONS	METHOD OF APPLICATION	BLENDS WELL WITH
Skin: Mature skin, wrinkles, scar tissue, wounds, eczema, psoriasis, acne, inflamed skin conditions, insect bites. Soothing to dry, irritated skin	Body or facial oil, body butter, aromatic gel, salve, unscented cleanser, cream or lotion	Calendula CO₂, Cape Chamomile, Carrot Seed, Cistus, Cypress, Frankincense, Helichrysum, Lavender, Lemon, Lemongrass, Petitgrain, Thyme ct. linalool, Yarrow
Psyche/emotions: Anxiety, tension, inability to focus, irritability, anger, frustration, feeling overwhelmed by stress or pressure. Supports reflection and introspection	Personal inhaler, roll-on, aromatic spritzer	Angelica Root, Cape Chamomile, Cistus, Frankincense, Grapefruit, Lavender, Lemon, Sweet Marjoram, Sweet Orange, Petitgrain, Pinyon Pine, Valerian, Yarrow, Ylang Ylang

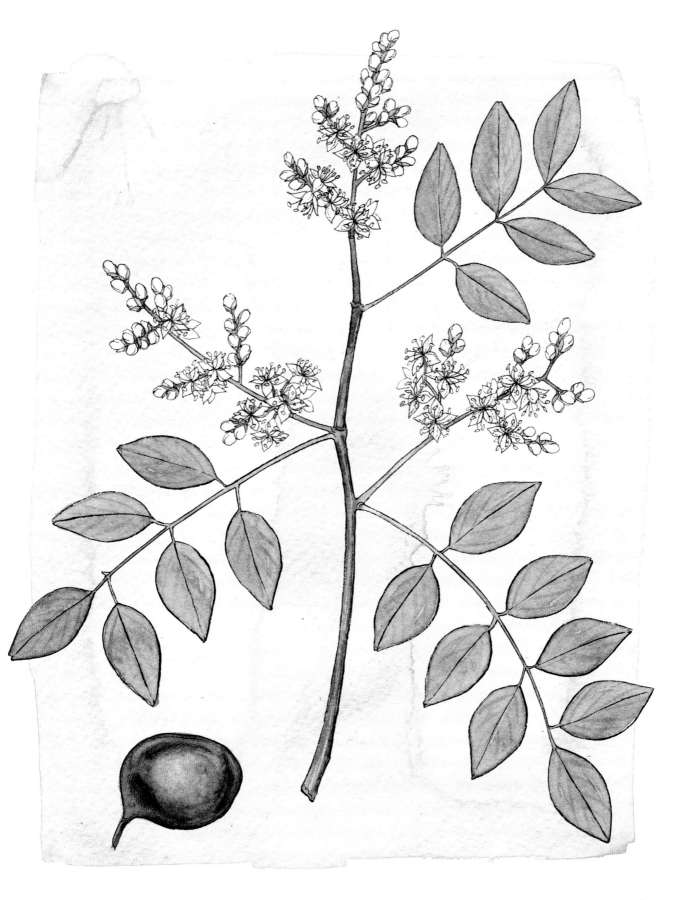

FRANKINCENSE

Frankincense (*Boswellia sacra* syn. *Boswellia carteri*, Burseraceae) essential oil is steam distilled using the resin of the frankincense tree.

SOURCE COUNTRIES: Somalia, India, North Africa, and Oman

CORE CHEMICAL COMPONENTS: α-pinene and d-limonene

DERMAL CAUTION: Potential skin sensitizer if the oil is oxidized. Avoid older oils and store correctly.

CONSERVATION: Not yet assessed

BLENDING WITH FRANKINCENSE

AROMA: Clean, fresh, earthy, woody

SYSTEM AFFINITY: Skin

BLENDS WELL WITH: Bergamot Mint, Black Pepper, Calendula CO2, Himalayan Cedarwood, Roman Chamomile, Cistus, Copaiba, Cypress, Blue Gum Eucalyptus, Goldenrod, Inula, Lavender, Lemon, Lemongrass, Lime, Mandarin, Melissa, Myrrh, Neroli, Niaouli, Sweet Orange, Patchouli, Scots Pine, Pinyon Pine, Rose, Hemlock Spruce

POTENTIAL SUBSTITUTIONS: Lavender, Myrrh, Cistus

THERAPEUTIC APPLICATIONS

INDICATIONS	METHOD OF APPLICATION	PAIRS WELL WITH
Skin: Mature skin, wrinkles, scar tissue, postoperative wound healing (once sutures are removed), eczema, acne, inflamed skin conditions, blackheads, hives. Soothing to dry, irritated skin	Unscented cream or lotion, salve, body butter, body or facial oil	Himalayan Cedarwood, Roman Chamomile, Cistus, Copaiba, Cypress, Lavender, Lemongrass, Melissa, Myrrh, Neroli, Niaouli, Patchouli, Rose
Respiratory system: Bronchitis, sinus congestion, asthma	Steam inhalation, personal inhaler, chest salve, nebulizing diffuser	Cypress, Blue Gum Eucalyptus, Goldenrod, Inula, Lemon, Niaouli, Scots Pine, Pinyon Pine, Hemlock Spruce
Psyche/emotions: Anxiety, tension, inability to focus. Meditative, supports reflection and introspection, healing on all levels of spirit and emotion, stills the mind, promotes spiritual consciousness and tranquility, soothes the spirit. A wonderful oil to demonstrate the mind-body connection	Personal inhaler, diffuser, nebulizing diffuser, roll-on, aromatic bath	Bergamot Mint, Himalayan Cedarwood, Roman Chamomile, Lavender, Lemon, Lime, Mandarin, Melissa, Myrrh, Neroli, Sweet Orange, Patchouli, Scots Pine, Pinyon Pine, Rose, Hemlock Spruce

LAVENDER

Considered the "mother of all essential oils," **Lavender** essential oil is steam distilled using the flowering tops and leaves of the lavender plant, *Lavandula angustifolia* (Lamiaceae family). It's sometimes called the one essential oil never to leave home without! It not only provides a spectrum of possible uses, it is considered an enhancer (an oil that boosts the therapeutic benefits of other oils) for just about all other essential oils.

SOURCE COUNTRIES: France, Bulgaria, China, India, South Africa, and the United States

CORE COMPONENTS: Linalool, linalyl acetate, lavandulyl acetate

DERMAL CAUTION: No known cautions

CONSERVATION: Least concern

BLENDING WITH LAVENDER

AROMA: Fresh, floral, sweet, herbaceous

SYSTEM AFFINITIES: Skin, all systems

BLENDS WELL WITH: Most essential oils

POTENTIAL SUBSTITUTIONS: Lavender has such a wide range of activity that is unique to it that it would be challenging to replace. We recommend choosing a substitution based upon what you are looking for the oil to do in the blend/formulation.

THERAPEUTIC APPLICATIONS

INDICATIONS	METHOD OF APPLICATION	PAIRS WELL WITH
Skin: Burns, scrapes, acne, athlete's foot, eczema, inflamed skin conditions, psoriasis, sunburn, itchy skin, insect bites	Gel, unscented cream or lotion, body or facial oil, foot bath, lip balm	See reference chart on page 198.
Reproductive system: Labor and delivery. Can help reduce severity of contractions (use with Clary Sage); helps in relieving menstrual cramps	Personal inhaler, diffuser, nebulizing diffuser, aromatic baths, roll-on	Basil ct. linalool, Clary Sage Sweet Fennel, Geranium, Jasmine Absolute, Lavender, Mandarin, Sweet Marjoram, Neroli, Petitgrain, Rose
Musculoskeletal system: Muscular aches and pains, arthritis, sprains, strains, growing pains, plantar fasciitis, tendonitis, shin splints, rheumatic conditions, joint pain and stiffness, bursitis	Body oil, salve, gel, roll-on, aromatic bath	Basil ct. linalool, Bergamot Mint, Black Pepper, Clove Bud, Ginger, Juniper Berry, Laurel, Sweet Marjoram, Peppermint, Rosemary ct. camphor or Rosemary ct. cineole, Wintergreen
Psyche/emotions: Irritability, mild depression, anxiety, hyperactivity, panic attacks, insomnia	Aromatic bath, personal inhaler, roll-on, diffuser, nebulizing diffuser, aromatic spritzer	Bergamot, Cardamom, German Chamomile, Roman Chamomile, Grapefruit, Lemon, Mandarin, Neroli, Sweet Orange, Petitgrain, Pinyon Pine, Rose, Ylang Ylang

LAVENDIN

Lavendin (*Lavandula x intermedia*, Lamiaceae) essential oil is steam distilled using the flowering tops of the lavendin plant. Lavendin is much loved for its soothing and calming properties while also being able to relieve muscular aches and pains or support wound healing.

SOURCE COUNTRY: France

CORE COMPONENTS: linalool, linalyl acetate

DERMAL CAUTION: No known contraindications or concerns

CONSERVATION: Not yet assessed

BLENDING WITH LAVENDIN

AROMA: Fresh, floral, sweet, herbaceous, camphoraceous

SYSTEM AFFINITIES: Skin, musculoskeletal, emotions

BLENDS WELL WITH: Calendula CO_2 Extract, Carrot Seed, Clary Sage, Frankincense, Helichrysum, Lavender, Sweet Marjoram, Mandarin, Neroli, Patchouli, Petitgrain, Rosemary ct. verbenone, Thyme ct. linalool

POTENTIAL SUBSTITUTIONS: Lavender, Frankincense

THERAPEUTIC APPLICATIONS

INDICATIONS	METHOD OF APPLICATION	BLENDS WELL WITH
Skin: Burns, bacterial skin infections, allergic skin reactions (combine with blue tansy), wound healing	Gel, unscented cream or lotion, salve, aromatic baths	Carrot Seed, Frankincense, Helichrysum, Lavender, Neroli, Petitgrain, Rosemary ct. verbenone
Psyche/emotions: Lethargy, insomnia, anxiety, depression, migraine, nervousness, sleep disorders. Relieves tension	Personal inhaler, diffuser, nebulizing diffuser, roll-on	Clary Sage, Frankincense, Lavender, Mandarin, Sweet Marjoram, Neroli, Patchouli, Petitgrain
Musculoskeletal system: Muscular stiffness, sprains, neuralgia	Gel, body oil, salve	Helichrysum, Sweet Marjoram, Lavender, Rosemary ct. verbenone

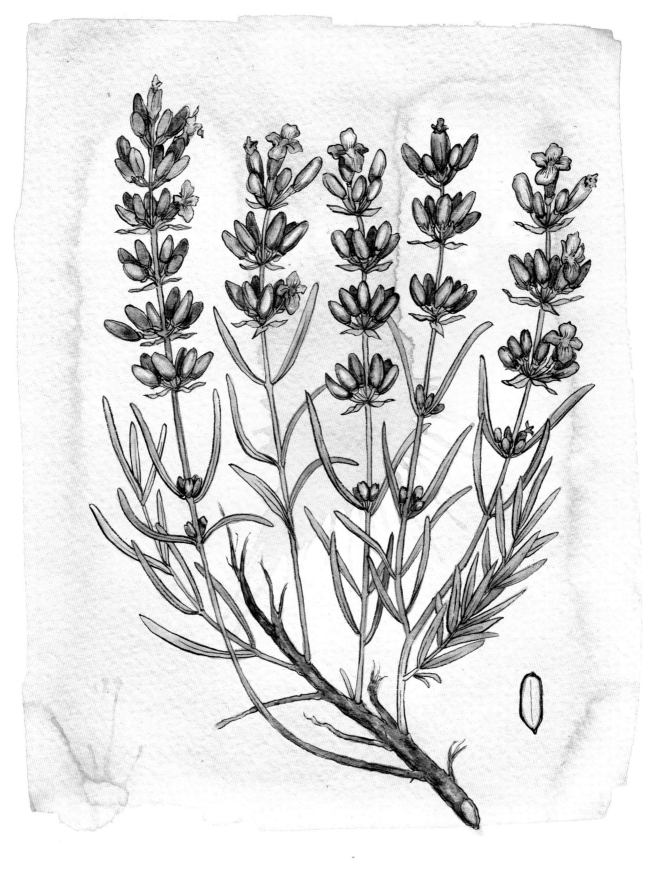

LEMON

Lemon (*Citrus limon*, Rutaceae) essential oil is expressed or steam distilled using lemon peel or zest. It can be used for uplifting emotions, reducing the impact of stress, supporting the body as it fights infection, and overall health and well-being. A must-have essential oil that pairs well with others.

SOURCE COUNTRIES: Italy, United States, Argentina, Italy (Sicily), and Greece (Cyprus)

CORE COMPONENTS: D-limonene, β-pinene, c-terpinene

DERMAL ALERT: Oxidized citrus essential oils such as lemon shouldn't be used in body care products for the skin, but can be used for cleaning products.

DERMAL CAUTION: Expressed lemon has a very low risk of being photosensitizing; distilled lemon is not phototoxic. Dilution rate for skin products is 12 to18 drops per ounce of carrier oil or base product.

CONSERVATION: Not defined

BLENDING WITH LEMON

AROMA: Sharp, citrus, refreshing

SYSTEM AFFINITIES: Digestive, circulatory

BLENDS WELL WITH: Basil ct. linalool, Celery Seed, Cinnamon Leaf, Clary Sage, Cypress, Blue Gum Eucalyptus, Douglas Fir, Fingerroot, Frankincense, Ginger, Goldenrod, Grapefruit, Juniper Berry, Katafray, Lavender, Lemongrass, Myrrh, Neroli, Niaouli, Palmarosa, Pink Pepper, Scots Pine, Pinyon Pine, Rosemary ct. cineole or Rosemary ct. camphor, Hemlock Spruce, Tea Tree

POTENTIAL SUBSTITUTIONS: Grapefruit, Sweet Orange

THERAPEUTIC APPLICATIONS

INDICATIONS	METHOD OF APPLICATION	PAIRS WELL WITH
Skin: Acne, premature aging skin (preventative), oily complexions, mouth ulcers, cellulite, rosacea, broken capillaries	Unscented cream or lotion, gel, body or facial oil	Celery Seed, Cypress, Frankincense, Lavender, Lemongrass, Myrrh, Neroli, Niaouli, Palmarosa, Tea Tree
Circulatory system: Poor circulation, capillary fragility, varicose veins	Salt scrub* *Do not use on varicose veins.	Celery Seed, Cypress, Grapefruit, Juniper Berry, Lemongrass, Rosemary ct. cineole
Musculoskeletal system: Muscular or joint aches and pains, arthritis, cellulite, rheumatism, joint swelling, gout	Body oil, gel, body salt scrub	Basil ct. linalool, Clary Sage, Ginger, Grapefruit, Juniper Berry, Katafray, Lavender, Lemongrass, Pinyon Pine, Rosemary ct. cineole or Rosemary ct. camphor, Hemlock Spruce
Psyche/emotions: Anxiety, depression, stress, anger/irritability	Personal inhaler, diffuser, nebulizing diffuser, salt inhaler	Basil ct. linalool, Clary Sage, Douglas Fir, Frankincense, Grapefruit, Lavender, Neroli, Pinyon Pine, Hemlock Spruce

NEROLI

Indigenous to Italy, **Neroli** (*Citrus aurantium* var. *amara*, Rutaceae) essential oil is steam distilled using the flowers of the bitter orange tree. It was named after the princess of Nerola in Italy, who used the perfumed oil to scent her gloves and bathwater.

SOURCE COUNTRIES: Australia, Madagascar, and New Caledonia

CORE COMPONENTS: D-limonene, linalool, linalyl acetate

SAFETY: No known contraindications

CONSERVATION: Not defined

BLENDING WITH NEROLI

AROMA: Sweet, floral

SYSTEM AFFINITIES: Skin, psyche/emotions

BLENDS WELL WITH: Angelica Root, Basil ct. linalool, Bergamot Mint, Calendula CO2, Celery Seed, Cistus, Copaiba, Clary Sage, Coriander Seed, Cypress, Fingerroot, Grapefruit, Lavender, Lemongrass, Mandarin, Myrrh, Sweet Orange, Palmarosa, Petitgrain, Pinyon Pine, Hemlock Spruce, Valerian, Ylang Ylang

POTENTIAL SUBSTITUTIONS: Jasmine, Petitgrain, Ylang Ylang

THERAPEUTIC APPLICATIONS

INDICATIONS	METHOD OF APPLICATION	PAIRS WELL WITH
Skin: Oily skin conditions, spider veins, stretch marks, wounds	Facial oil, cream, lotion, body butter	Calendula CO2, Cistus, Copaiba, Cypress, Lavender, Myrrh, Palmarosa, Petitgrain
Reproductive system: PMS, menopause, pregnancy and labor, sexual frigidity, anxiety during labor and childbirth, low libido	Personal inhaler, body oil, roll-on	Basil ct. linalool, Lavender, Mandarin, Sweet Orange, Petitgrain, Ylang Ylang
Psyche/emotions: Depression, anxiety, heartache, agitation, tachycardia, insomnia, stress and stress-related conditions, panic attacks, hot, agitated conditions of the heart characterized by restlessness	Personal inhaler, roll-on, body oil, cream, lotion, facial oil, aromatic bath	Angelica Root, Basil ct. linalool, Bergamot Mint, Coriander Seed, Grapefruit, Mandarin, Myrrh, Sweet Orange, Petitgrain, Pinyon Pine, Valerian, Ylang Ylang

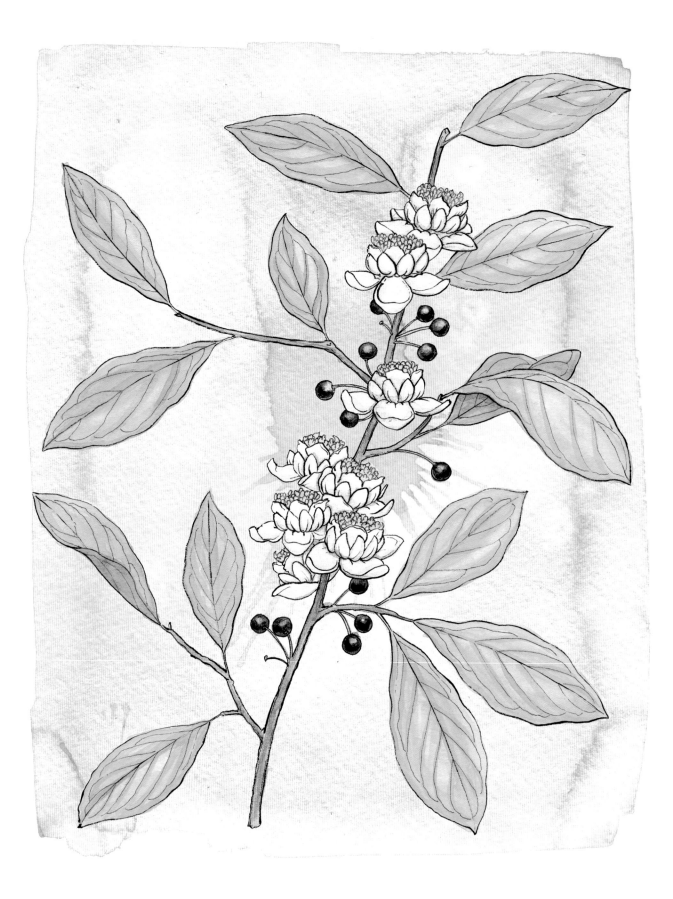

MAY CHANG

May Chang (*Litsea cubeba*, Lauraceae) essential oil is steam distilled using the ripe fruit.

SOURCE COUNTRY: China

CORE COMPONENTS: Geranial, neral, limonene, linalool

DERMAL CAUTION: Recommended dilution to avoid skin irritation, 1 drop per one teaspoon of carrier oil or other base (e.g., unscented cream or lotion)

CONSERVATION: Not yet assessed

BLENDING WITH MAY CHANG

AROMA: Grass-like with lemony notes, fresh and light yet sharp

SYSTEM AFFINITIES: Skin

BLENDS WELL WITH: Bergamot, Cape Chamomile, Cistus, Clove Bud, Frankincense, Geranium, Ginger, Grapefruit, Laurel, Lavender, Lemon, Lemongrass, Sweet Marjoram, Sweet Orange, Petitgrain

POTENTIAL SUBSTITUTIONS: Lemongrass

THERAPEUTIC APPLICATIONS

INDICATIONS	METHOD OF APPLICATION	PAIRS WELL WITH:
Skin: Mild infections, acne, oily skin	Facial oil, body or facial cleanser	Cape Chamomile, Cistus, Frankincense, Lavender, Lemon, Sweet Marjoram
Musculoskeletal system: Muscular aches and pains, arthritis, rheumatic pain	Body oil, salve, gel	Clove Bud, Ginger, Grapefruit, Laurel, Lavender, Lemon, Lemongrass, Sweet Marjoram
Psyche/emotions: Stress, anxiety, overwhelmed, nervousness, insecurity, low self esteem	Personal inhaler, diffuser, roll-on	Bergamot, Cape Chamomile, Frankincense, Geranium, Grapefruit, Lavender, Lemon, Sweet Marjoram, Sweet Orange, Petitgrain

PALMAROSA

Palmarosa (*Cymbopogon martinii*, Poaceae) essential oil is steam distilled using the palmarosa grass. With its strong affinity to the skin, palmarosa supports the skin's health by promoting cellular rejuvenation and defends against bacterial or fungal infections.

SOURCE COUNTRIES: India, Brazil, South Africa, and Nepal

CORE COMPONENTS: Geraniol

SAFETY: No known contraindications

CONSERVATION: Not defined

BLENDING WITH PALMAROSA

AROMA: Sweet, floral, rosy

SYSTEM AFFINITIES: Skin

BLENDS WELL WITH: Carrot Seed, Himalayan Cedarwood, Clove, Lavender, Laurel, Niaouli, Neroli, Rosemary ct. verbenone, Thyme ct. linalool

POTENTIAL SUBSTITUTIONS: Carrot Seed + Lavender, Neroli

THERAPEUTIC APPLICATIONS

INDICATIONS	METHOD OF APPLICATION	PAIRS WELL WITH
Skin: Acne, dry skin, mature skin, fungal infections, dermatitis, eczema (dry and weeping), psoriasis, boils, wounds, cuts, wrinkles, itchy skin, broken capillaries	Cleanser, cream or lotion, gel, body oil, salve, salt scrub Used in homemade underarm deodorant to prevent odor	Carrot Seed, Himalayan Cedarwood, Lavender, Niaouli, Neroli, Rosemary ct. verbenone, Thyme ct. linalool
Psyche/emotions: Restlessness, anxiety, tension, nervous exhaustion, heartache, irritability, stress	Personal inhaler, diffuser, roller ball	Carrot Seed, Himalayan Cedarwood, Lavender, Neroli

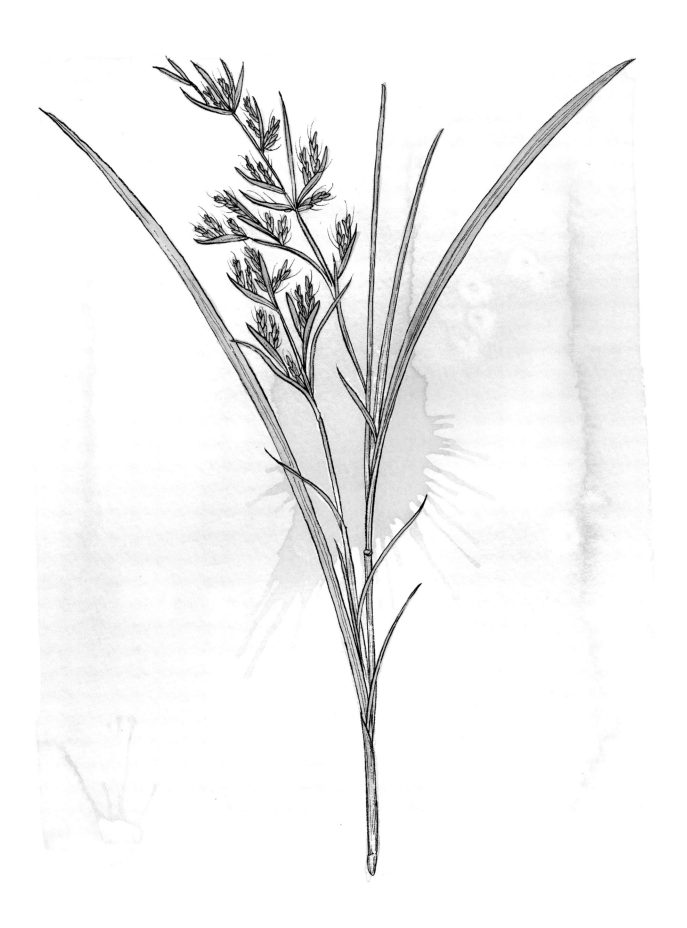

PATCHOULI

Patchouli (*Pogostemon cablin*, Lamiaceae) essential oil is steam distilled using dried patchouli leaves. This is one of those essential oils people seem to either love or hate. It offers wonderful benefits for the skin due to its slightly astringent-like activity and skin soothing properties. Its aroma nourishes and calms the spirits (at least, it does if you love it!)

SOURCE COUNTRIES: Indonesia, India, China, and Brazil

CORE COMPONENTS: Patchouli alcohol

SAFETY: No known contraindications

CONSERVATION: Not yet assessed

BLENDING WITH PATCHOULI

AROMA: Strong, musty, earthy, dry

SYSTEM AFFINITIES: Skin

BLENDS WELL WITH: Angelica Root, Bergamot, Black Pepper, Cardamom, Cinnamon Leaf, Cistus, Clary Sage, Cypress, Geranium, Ginger, Grapefruit, Lavender, Lemongrass, Mandarin, Sweet Orange, Peppermint, Rose, Blue Tansy, Valerian

POTENTIAL SUBSTITUTIONS: Vetiver, Cypress

THERAPEUTIC APPLICATIONS

INDICATIONS	METHOD OF APPLICATION	PAIRS WELL WITH
Skin: Aging or sagging skin, itchy or inflamed skin conditions, acne, athlete's foot, cracked or chapped skin, eczema (weeping), wrinkles, irritated skin conditions, sores, allergic inflammation, cellulite	Facial or body oil, body butter, aromatic gel, salves, salt scrubs	Cistus, Cypress, Geranium, Grapefruit, Lavender, Sweet Orange, Rose, Blue Tansy
Reproductive system: Frigidity, menstrual cramps, reduced or lack of sex drive, impotence	Personal inhaler, body oil, diffuser, abdominal oil	Bergamot, Black Pepper, Cardamom, Cinnamon Leaf, Clary Sage, Geranium, Grapefruit, Lavender, Mandarin, Sweet Orange, Rose
Psyche/emotions: Anxiety, depression, confusion, poor concentration, mood swings, hyperactivity, anxiety, feelings of being overwhelmed	Body oil, body butter, salve (used like perfume), aromatic baths, unscented cream/lotions, personal inhalers, aromatic spritzer	Angelica Root, Bergamot, Black Pepper, Clary Sage, Cypress, Geranium, Grapefruit, Lavender, Mandarin, Sweet Orange, Rose, Valerian
General: Useful in mosquito repellents, serves to hold other essential oils (as a base or fixative) so insect repellants and perfumes last longer and are more effective	Aromatic spritzer	Himalayan Cedarwood, Geranium, Lemongrass, Peppermint

YARROW

Yarrow (*Achillea millefolium*, Asteraceae) essential oil is steam distilled using the flowering yarrow plant (feathery leaves and flowers). Often, but not always, it is a rich blue essential oil. Yarrow is much loved for its wound healing and anti-inflammatory activity.

SOURCE COUNTRY: France

CORE COMPONENTS: Monoterpenes: sabinene and β-pinene. Sesquiterpenes: β-caryophyllene and germacrene D. The chemistry of yarrow is quite variable, with some containing chamazulene (blue color) and others containing only a small to no amount of chamazulene (light blue to light yellow).

SAFETY: No known cautions

CONSERVATION: Least concern

BLENDING WITH YARROW

AROMA: Sweet, spicy, warm, fresh

SYSTEM AFFINITIES: Skin

BLENDS WELL WITH: Calendula CO2, Cape Chamomile, German Chamomile, Roman Chamomile, Carrot Seed, Clary Sage, Cistus, Frankincense, Lavender, Neroli, Niaouli, Rosemary ct. verbenone,

POTENTIAL SUBSTITUTIONS: Lavender, German Chamomile, Cape Chamomile

THERAPEUTIC APPLICATIONS

INDICATIONS	METHOD OF APPLICATION	PAIRS WELL WITH
Skin: Inflamed conditions, razor burn, dermatitis, acne, eczema, burns, cuts, rashes, scars, wounds, varicose veins, bruises. Tones the skin, slows bleeding from trauma, preventative to premature aging	Cream, facial oil, cleanser, aromatic bath	Cape Chamomile, Frankincense, Lavender, Calendula CO2, Cistus, German Chamomile, Carrot Seed
Musculoskeletal system: Arthritis, rheumatism, aches and pains, stiffness, cramps, tendinitis	Body oil, gel, salve, lotion	Clary Sage, Cape Chamomile, Lavender, Rosemary ct. cineole or Rosemary ct. camphor
Psyche/emotions: Nervous tension, irritability, neuralgia, insomnia, nervousness, anxiety, depression, restlessness	Body butter, personal inhaler, aromatic baths, diffuser	Cape Chamomile, Frankincense, Lavender, German Chamomile

PETITGRAIN

Petitgrain (*Citrus aurantium* var. *amara*, Rutaceae) essential oil is steam distilled using the leaves of the bitter orange tree. Much loved for its stress-relieving aroma, petitgrain is used almost exclusively for emotional well-being and skin care.

SOURCE COUNTRY: Italy

CORE CHEMICAL COMPONENTS: Linalool, linalyl acetate, α-terpineol, geraniol and geranyl acetate

DERMAL CAUTION: No known cautions or contraindications

CONSERVATION: Not defined

BLENDING WITH PETITGRAIN

AROMA: Woody, dry, floral, light

SYSTEM AFFINITIES: Nervous, psyche/emotions, skin

BLENDS WELL WITH: Cardamom, Cypress, Grapefruit, Lavender, Lemon, Mandarin, Sweet Marjoram, Neroli, Sweet Orange, Patchouli, Rose

POTENTIAL SUBSTITUTIONS: Lavender, Neroli, Bitter Orange

THERAPEUTIC APPLICATIONS

INDICATIONS	METHOD OF APPLICATION	PAIRS WELL WITH
Skin: Acne, inflamed skin (supports neroli and lavender), eczema, boils. A mild astringent, good for oily as well as dry skin, toning, wound healing	Cleanser, gel, unscented cream	Cypress, Grapefruit, Lavender, Lemon, Neroli, Patchouli, Rose
Reproductive system: Menstrual cramps, PMS, emotions associated with menopause. Could be used during childbirth as a pleasant, relaxing aroma	Personal inhaler, abdominal oil, diffuser, nebulizing diffuser	Cardamom, Cypress, Grapefruit, Lavender, Mandarin, Sweet Marjoram, Neroli, Sweet Orange, Patchouli, Rose
Psyche/emotions: Anxiety, tension, nervousness, irritation, insomnia, mental fatigue, mild depression, heart palpitations from anxiety or stress, agitation, psychological stress	Personal inhaler, diffuser, roller ball, body oil, salt scrub, body butter	Cardamom, Cypress, Grapefruit, Lavender, Lemon, Mandarin, Sweet Marjoram, Neroli, Sweet Orange, Patchouli, Rose

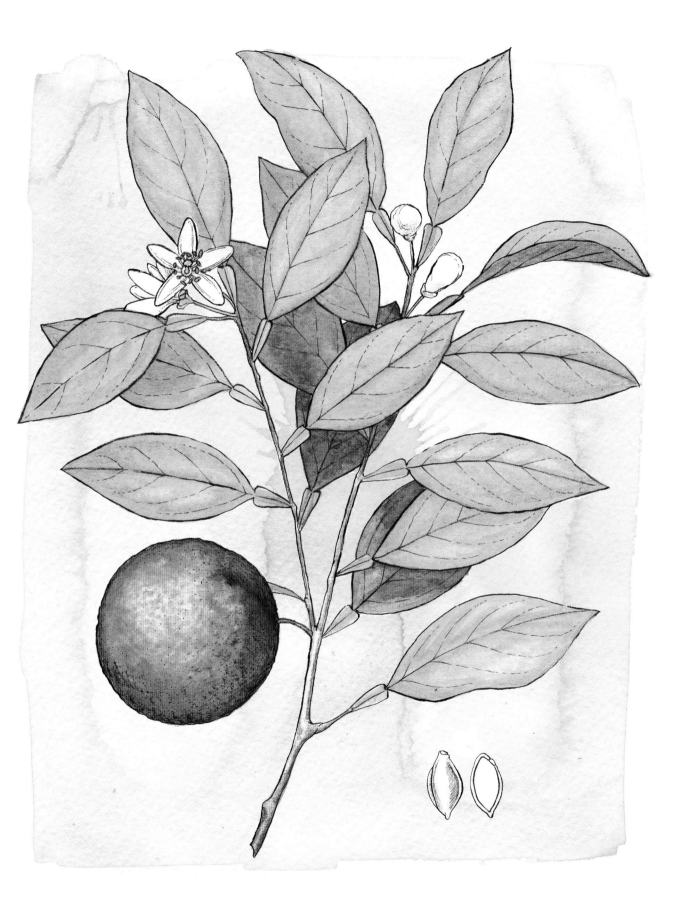

SANDALWOOD

Sandalwood (*Santalum album*, Santalaceae) essential oil is steam distilled using the heartwood of the tree trunk. Much loved for its gentle transcendent aroma, sandalwood has a strong affinity to the skin which it will soothe, protect, and nourish.

SOURCE COUNTRIES: India, New Caledonia, Hawaii, and Australia

CORE COMPONENTS: α-santalol, β-santalol, and cis-lanceol

SAFETY: No known contraindications or cautions

CONSERVATION: Vulnerable

BLENDING WITH SANDALWOOD

AROMA: Balsamic, woody, slightly sweet and musky

SYSTEM AFFINITIES: Skin

BLENDS WELL WITH: Clary Sage, Copaiba, Frankincense, Geranium, Lavender, Lemon, Mandarin, Rose

POTENTIAL SUBSTITUTIONS: Frankincense

THERAPEUTIC APPLICATIONS

INDICATIONS	METHOD OF APPLICATION	PAIRS WELL WITH:
Skin: Acne, dry, cracked and/or chapped skin, dry eczema, razor/shaving rash, oily skin, itchy or inflamed skin, mature or aging skin, varicose veins, cold sores, protective against damage from the sun	Unscented cream or lotion, facial or body oil, salve, body butter	Copaiba, Frankincense, Lavender, Rose
Psyche/emotions: insomnia, nervous tension, stress, depression, anger, stress-related conditions, agitation	Personal inhaler, roll-on	Clary Sage, Frankincense, Geranium, Lavender, Lemon, Mandarin, Rose

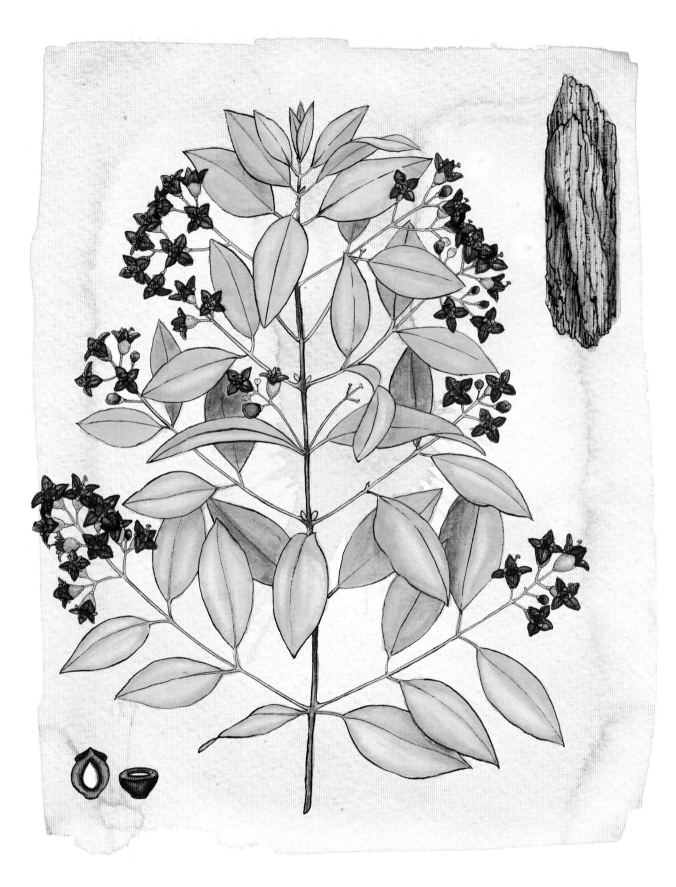

THYME

SKIN SYSTEM

Thyme (*Thymus vulgaris*, Lamiaceae) essential oil has several chemotypes available. In this book we will focus on two of the main thyme chemotypes we find ourselves using on a regular basis.

THYME CT. LINALOOL

SOURCE COUNTRY: France

CORE COMPONENT: 1,8 cineole, *a*-pinene, camphor, and β-caryophyllene

SAFETY: No known cautions or contraindications

CONSERVATION: Not defined

BLENDING WITH THYME CT. LINALOOL

AROMA: Sweet, slightly floral, soft herbaceous

SYSTEM AFFINITY: Skin

BLENDS WELL WITH: Anise, Calendula CO_2, Roman Chamomile, Cinnamon Leaf, Coriander

POTENTIAL SUBSTITUTIONS: Niaouli

THERAPEUTIC APPLICATIONS

INDICATIONS	METHOD OF APPLICATION	PAIRS WELL WITH
Skin: Skin infections, acne	Gel, unscented cream or lotion, facial cleanser	Carrot Seed, Roman Chamomile, Cinnamon Leaf, Copaiba, Cypress
Respiratory system: Lowered immunity, respiratory infections	Salve, steam inhalation	Cardamom, Cypress, Blue Gum Eucalyptus, Inula, Laurel, Niaouli
Musculoskeletal system: Muscular aches and pains, cramps, spasms, and rheumatic pain	Salve, unscented cream or lotion, body oil	Basil ct. linalool, Bergamot Mint, Black Pepper, Clary Sage, Lavender

THYME CT. THYMOL

SOURCE COUNTRY: France

CORE COMPONENT: 1,8 cineole, α-pinene, camphor, and β-caryophyllene

DERMAL CAUTION: Potential mucus membrane irritant. Avoid use in baths or undiluted to avoid skin irritation.

CONSERVATION: Least concerned

BLENDING WITH THYME CT. THYMOL

AROMA: Sharp, herbaceous

SYSTEM AFFINITIES: Respiratory, digestive

BLENDS WELL WITH: Anise, Roman Chamomile, Cinnamon Leaf, Cypress, Blue Gum Eucalyptus, Grapefruit, Inula, Laurel, Green Myrtle, Niaouli, Plai, Thyme ct. linalool

POTENTIAL SUBSTITUTIONS: Niaouli, Thyme ct. linalool

THERAPEUTIC APPLICATIONS

INDICATIONS	METHOD OF APPLICATION	PAIRS WELL WITH
Respiratory system: Bronchitis, sinusitis, respiratory infections, coughs, colds, flu. Powerful anti-infectious essential oil	Steam inhalation, personal inhaler, chest salve, chest oil	Anise, Cinnamon Leaf, Cypress, Blue Gum Eucalyptus, Inula, Laurel, Green Myrtle, Plai, Thyme ct. linalool

PART IV

Methods of Use (Application)

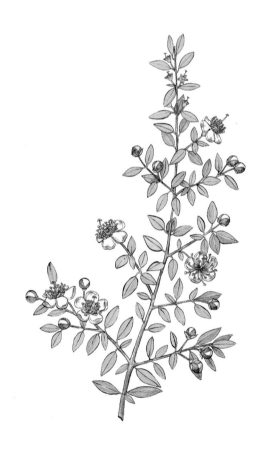

CHAPTER SIX

EXPANDING YOUR APOTHECARY

BEFORE WE DIVE into making body care products, we'll need to expand your apothecary with a few other botanical ingredients. As we discussed in chapter 3, aromatherapy body care products are made up of essential oils and some type of base, such as a carrier oil and/or herbal oil, an unscented cream or lotion, or a gel or salve. The following chart outlines the ingredients that each body care product covered in this book may contain. The lowercase x stands for optional or dependent upon the needs of product making.

	CO	HO	HY	WX	BT	AO
Body and Facial Oils	X	X				X
Roll-On (aka Roller Balls)	X	X				
Body Butters	X	X			X	X
Aromatic Gels	X	X	X			
Salves	X	X		X	X	X
Lip Balm	X	X		X	X	
Salt Scrubs	X	X				

Key to Codes

CO Carrier oil (includes vegetable oils and specialty seed oils, e.g., rosehip seed, borage)

HO Herbal oils (e.g., Calendula, St. John's Wort, Arnica)

HY Hydrosol(s)

WX Wax

BT Butter

AO Antioxidant

You can choose to make a body care product for its therapeutic benefits (e.g., a respiratory salve or salve to reduce inflamed skin conditions) or simply for the beauty and emotional support the aromatics provide (e.g., salve with rose, sweet orange, and patchouli used as a perfume).

Now let's add to your apothecary by understanding the ingredients needed to make various body care products.

CARRIER OILS

Carrier oils, also commonly referred to as vegetable oils, are expeller pressed (using a type of pressing machine that extracts the oil) from seeds, nuts, and whole fruits. They are called "carrier" oils because they help dilute and carry the essential oils onto the skin.

On their own, carrier oils have incredible therapeutic benefits that support the skin's health and vitality. Carrier oils contain a rich array of fat-soluble vitamins, fatty acids, and essential fatty acids that not only help nourish the skin, but also protect the skin's barrier function, protect and repair the skin from damage (be it from the sun or free radicals), and prevent transepidermal water loss (TEWL). Carrier oils can also support the tone, elasticity, shape, and resiliency of the skin.

Let's have a quick look at some of the more important fat-soluble vitamins and fatty acids found in carrier oils.

- **Vitamin E**, also known as tocopherols, is an important and potent antioxidant, which means that it prevents cell damage from the destructive elements of free radicals.

- **Vitamin A** is thought to support collagen synthesis and to support the health of the skin as it naturally ages or if it has been damaged from sun exposure.

THE NEED FOR AN ANTIOXIDANT

Carrier oils that are rich in essential fatty acids—that includes borage seed oil, rosehip seed oil, evening primrose oils, flax seed oil, and safflower and sunflower oils—are very unstable and can easily oxidize if exposed to oxygen, heat, and light. When using these carriers in a body care product, we encourage you to add in an antioxidant such as vitamin E, mixed tocopherols, or rosemary CO_2 extract. This will help stabilize the above carrier oils and extend their shelf life for up to 6 to 12 months.

- **Beta-carotene**, a precursor to vitamin A, is found in carriers that tend to be a rich orange color, such as sea buckthorn CO_2 extract and palm kernel oil. Beta-carotene protects the skin from free-radical damage as well as damage from the sun.

- **Essential fatty acids**, such as linoleic and linolenic acid, are fatty acids the body cannot make on its own. We need to apply them to our skin or take them into our body through our diet. Deficiency in essential fatty acids in the skin alters the barrier function of the skin and can lead to excessive dryness (from water loss), scaliness, redness, and other inflamed skin conditions. Carrier oils rich in essential fatty acids include borage, rosehip seed oil, evening primrose oil, flax seed oil, and safflower and sunflower oils (rich in linoleic acid).

Carrier Oils and Their Properties

The following chart provides information on a variety of carrier oils. Our favorite carrier oils and the ones we tend to use the most are: jojoba oil, sesame seed oil, and sunflower seed oil. These three carriers are readily available, relatively inexpensive, and can be used at 100 percent.

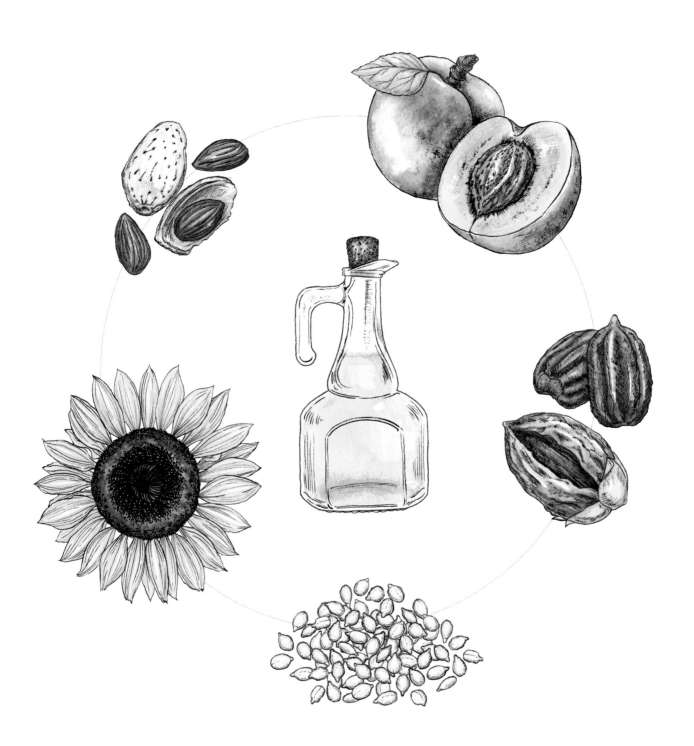

CARRIER OIL	PROPERTIES

AVOCADO OIL
Persea americana

Shelf Life: Up to 12 months. Can add mixed tocopherols or vitamin E to elongate shelf life: 0.04% to 1.0%.

Avocado oil offers powerful revitalizing and cell regenerative activity. Avocado is a wonderful emollient with great penetration. It's indicated specifically for maturing skin and dry skin. Post-menopausal skin, dry, dehydrated, fragile, or mature skin, and premature aging symptoms would all benefit from avocado oil.

Use: 10 to 15% dilution of the total carrier oil amount

BAOBAB OIL
Adansonia digitata

Shelf Life: 2 to 4 years dependent upon the conditions of storage. Extremely stable oil.

Baobab oil is a heavier oil than most other carrier oils, with great emollient qualities for the skin supporting the skins' barrier function and lipid matrix while preventing water loss.

Use: 25 to 100% dilution of the total carrier oil amount

BORAGE SEED OIL
Borago officinalis

Shelf Life: Once opened, up to 6 to 9 months dependent upon the conditions of storage.

Borage seed oil and Evening primrose oil are used for preventing premature aging of the skin as well as for regenerative skin care. Both oils also reduce inflammation and are used for psoriasis, eczema, and atopic dermatitis.

Use: 10 to 25% dilution of the total carrier oil amount

EVENING PRIMROSE OIL
Oenothera biennis

Shelf Life: Once opened, up to 12 months dependent upon the conditions of storage.

JOJOBA OIL
Simmondsia chinensis

Shelf Life: Once opened, up to 12 to 24 months dependent upon the conditions of storage.

What's most fascinating about this oil is that its molecular structure resembles a liquid wax rather than a lipid-rich oil. Because of its chemical composition, our skin finds it familiar to our own sebum, and subsequently it is quite effective when applied to soothe inflammation, support resiliency, and bring the skin back into balance. Jojoba helps oily skin, particularly if pores are clogged and/or inflamed. It's fast absorbing and stable.

Jojoba is highly versatile and can be a central ingredient in a wide array of skin and body care products. It is quite lovely when infused with vanilla beans. There are a lot of recipes on the internet.

NEEM OIL
Azadirachta indica

Shelf Life: Once opened, up to 6 to 9 months dependent upon the conditions of storage.

Native to India, Neem oil has a very potent pungent diffusive aroma. The oil shines in its ability to address dandruff, dry itchy scalps, and dry, damaged hair. Neem oil is also used in body care products for acne, eczema, foot fungus, and oily skin.

Neem oil also has mosquito-repellent qualities.

Use: 10 to 100% dilution of the total carrier oil amount

CARRIER OIL	PROPERTIES
POMEGRANATE OIL AND CO₂ TOTAL EXTRACT *Punica granatum* **Shelf Life:** Once opened, up to 6 to 9 months dependent upon the conditions of storage.	Pomegranate oil and CO_2 total extract soothes dermal inflammations such as acne, sunburn, psoriasis, and rosacea. It supports cellular regeneration, is a great antioxidant, improves skin elasticity, revitalizes prematurely aging or sun damaged skin, and is an incredibly beneficial emollient for dry skin conditions. **Carrier oil:** 10 to15% dilution of the total carrier oil amount **CO₂ total extract:** 1 to 15%
ROSEHIP SEED OIL AND CO₂ TOTAL EXTRACT *Rosa canina* or *Rosa rubignosa* **Shelf Life:** Once opened, up to 6 to 9 months dependent upon the conditions of storage.	Rosehip seed oil and CO_2 total extract are most often used for supporting cellular rejuvenation and preventing premature aging of the skin. Either can be added to body care formulations for wound healing, to reduce age spots, and for regenerative skin care (tissue regeneration). Post-menopausal, dry, dehydrated, fragile, mature, and prematurely aging skin would all benefit from rosehip seed oil and total CO_2 extract. **Carrier oil:** 10 to 50% dilution of the total carrier oil amount **CO₂ total extract:** 1 to 15%
SEA BUCKTHORN OIL *Hippophae rhamnoides* **Shelf Life:** Once opened, up to 6 to 9 months dependent upon the conditions of storage.	Sea buckthorn's vibrant orange colored carrier oil and CO_2 total extract are used to support healing of the skin, reduce inflammation with conditions such as eczema or psoriasis. This oil supports wound healing, slow or poorly healing wounds, and healing the skin from sun damage. **Carrier oil:** 5 to 10% dilution of the total carrier oil amount **CO₂ total extract:** 1 to 15% **Note:** Due to sea buckthorn's rich orange color, it can stain clothing and other material it comes into contact with. Rinse material in cold soapy water immediately to remove oil.
SESAME OIL *Sesamum indicum* **Shelf Life:** Up to 24 months. Sesame is one of the oils most resistant to oxidation because it contains the powerful natural antioxidants sesamolin and sesamin.	Sesame is also used to protect our skin from free-radical damage, and it strengthens the resiliency of our skin's barrier function with its trace vitamins and minerals. It has an oilier feel to the skin than jojoba and a very slight sesame-like aroma.
SUNFLOWER OIL *Helianthus annuus* **Shelf Life:** Once opened, up to 12 months dependent upon the conditions of storage.	Sunflower oil serves as a base oil that readily receives other more therapeutic carriers such as rosehip seed, calendula herbal oil, and pomegranate seed oil. **Note:** Sunflower is available as both an oleic-rich and linoleic-rich oil. Here we are discussing the use of the oleic-rich sunflower oil, which is most commonly available due to its stability even when exposed to heat.

CARRIER OIL	PROPERTIES
TAMANU OIL *Calophyllum inophyllum* **Shelf Life:** Once opened, up to 6 to 9 months dependent upon the conditions of storage.	Tamanu oil is a rich, aromatic carrier oil with a wide range of applications, many of which are based upon its traditional uses. Native to Southeast Asia, the tamanu tree is also found in Thailand, Vietnam, Myanmar, Malaysia, South India, and Sri Lanka. Tamanu is cell regenerative, wound healing, supportive to healthy scar tissue formation, and anti-inflammatory. It is also incredibly beneficial for dry/scaly skin conditions (e.g., psoriasis). **Use:** 10 to 100% dilution of the total carrier oil amount

HERBAL OILS

An herbal oil is made by combining plant material (e.g., dried calendula flowers) with a vegetable oil, typically extra virgin olive oil or oleic-rich sunflower oil, and allowing the plant material to soak in the oil for up to 3 months. During that time, the vegetable oil absorbs fat-soluble components from the plant material, many of which have therapeutic activity beneficial to the skin, muscles, and joints.

One of the herbal oils most commonly used in aromatherapy products is **CALENDULA** (*Calendula officinalis*). Calendula herbal oil soothes dry or inflamed skin, and it supports healing of mild burns, insect bites, and wounds. Calendula herbal oil also simply supports the health of the skin and can be used in facial oils, creams, lotions, and even gels.

ST. JOHN'S WORT (*Hypericum perforatum*) herbal oil is used in body care products such as gels or salves for insect bites, bruises, muscle pain, and inflamed skin conditions. St. John's wort helps reduce inflammation and relieve pain.

ARNICA (*Arnica montana*) herbal oil is used to relieve pain, support microcirculation, and reduce inflammation. Arnica herbal oil is used in body oils, salves, and homemade creams and lotions (designed for application to a localized area, e.g., the knees or wrists). Arnica oil is used for bruises, arthritis, bursitis, myalgia, sprains and strains, joint stiffness, and varicose veins. Safety note: Arnica herbal oil should not be applied to broken or damaged skin.

PLANT-DERIVED BUTTERS

Butters provide a nutrient-dense component to essential oil-focused skin care recipes indicated for damaged, weakened, and stressed skin. Butters are used in lip balms and body butters in this book. However, you may also see them used in homemade cream and lotion recipes. Butters such as shea, mango, and illipe have a remarkable capacity to heal tissue, soften the skin, strengthen the skin's barrier function, and prevent trans-epidermal water loss, thus preventing or healing dry skin.

The two most commonly used plant-based butters for aromatherapy body care products are shea butter and cocoa butter. They're used for slightly different purposes. Let's explore.

SHEA BUTTER (*Vitellaria paradoxa* (syn. *Butyrospermum parkii*)), extracted from the African shea nut tree, is softer to the touch than cocoa butter, and shares many of its therapeutic benefits. Shea butter softens and soothes dry, damaged skin and can relieve skin irritation. It can support tissue regeneration and resiliency. However, shea butter is

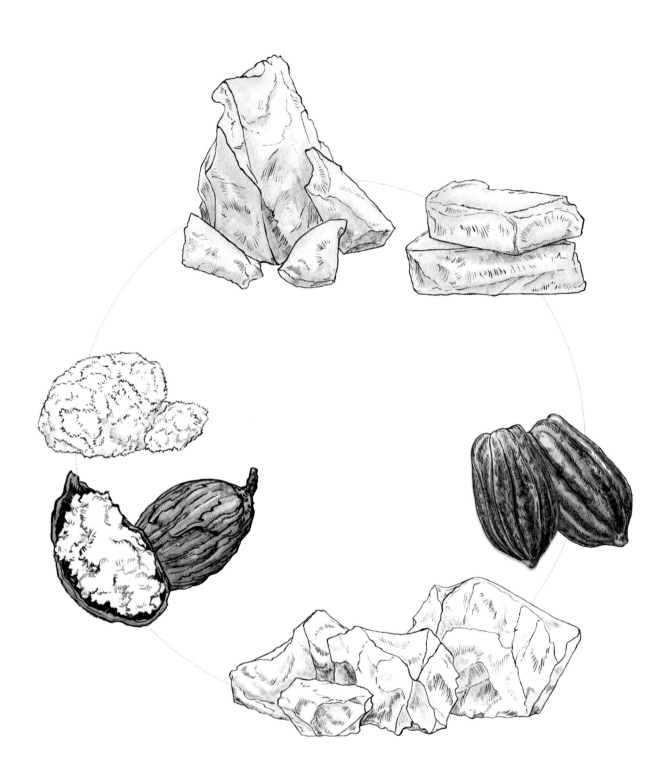

commonly used in and of itself for making whipped or regular body butters. Cocoa butter could not be used by itself to make a body butter, but it can be added in smaller amounts to support the therapeutic benefits of the butter. Unrefined shea butter is light to darker yellow in color and has a nutty, earthy aroma. Shea butter is used in body butters, lip balms, body balms, and at times, salves. It can be used up to 25 to 100 percent of a body butter or in a homemade cream or lotion. The shelf life of shea butter is 12 to 24 months when stored correctly.

COCOA BUTTER (*Theobroma cacao*) is the natural fatty byproduct of making chocolate from cocoa beans. Cocoa butter is used in lip balms, body butters, and homemade creams and lotions, and will harden in any product made with it. Due to its thickening/hardening nature, cocoa butter is used in low amounts. It can support the skin's health and prevent water loss—hence the reason why it is used in lip balms! It is recommended to use about 20 to 35 percent of the total recipe/formulation for body butters.

Unrefined cocoa butter smells strongly of chocolate, and it can often overpower the aromas of essential oils that are blended into it. We recommend choosing essential oils that smell good paired with the light scent of chocolate. Cocoa butter can last up to 2 to 5 years when stored properly. Keep away from heat, sunlight, and air. Note: Avoid over-heating cocoa butter. Over-heating or heating for too long breaks chemical bonds within the cocoa butter, resulting in its inability to harden again.

WAXES

For aromatherapy body care products, there are two core waxes to choose from: beeswax and a vegan alternative, candelilla wax. Wax is used in lip balms, salves, and homemade creams and lotions. It is used to thicken the product and is typically used at between 10 percent and 25 percent of the total recipe, depending on the product being made.

BEESWAX is typically a rich golden color, but it can vary depending on the propolis and colors within the pollen bees carry back to the hive. Beeswax has a beautiful sweet, honey-like aroma, which it imparts gently to the body care products that contain it. Please note: Bees and other pollinating insects face challenges in the ecosystems in which they play an essential role. If and when possible, purchase your beeswax from a local beekeeper, who uses healthy, sustainable practices.

CANDELILLA WAX is derived from the leaves of the small candelilla shrub, *Euphorbia cerifera* and *Euphorbia antisyphilitica*, which is native to northern Mexico and the southwestern United States. It is a yellowish-brown color and, like beeswax, is lightly aromatic. Candelilla wax is typically used at 10 to 12 percent of the total recipe. See page **164** for a recipe for a lip balm made with candelilla wax.

HYDROSOLS: AROMATIC WATERS

Hydrosols, also known as hydrolats, are one of the products of the distillation process. Hydrosols are quickly becoming much beloved for their gentle yet exceptional benefits for the skin and on emotional well-being. Artisan distillers all over the world are producing small batch hydrosols from ethically wild-crafted indigenous plants or lovingly cultivated plants grown for hydrosol distillation. There's never been a better time to explore these remarkable healing waters.

Hydrosols can soothe irritation, clean away bacteria and microbes from a cut or injury, reduce inflammation, support wound healing, soothe a sunburn, soothe irritated skin, and be used in gels for the skin, muscular aches and pains, or varicose veins.

Hydrosols can be used in baths, aromatic spritzers, homemade creams and lotions, and cleansers. They can also be used as toners for gentle skin care.

How much hydrosol to use?

- **Baths**

  ▷ Infants: 1 teaspoon (5 ml) of chosen hydrosol to an infant bathtub

  ▷ Children 2 to 6 years: 1 teaspoon (5 ml) of hydrosol per year of age, up to a maximum of 2 to 8 teaspoons (10 to 40 ml)

  ▷ 7 years and above and adults: 1 to 9 ounces (30 to 250 ml) per tub

- **Foot bath** (ages 7 years and above): 2 to 4 tablespoons (30 to 60 ml)

- **Aromatic Spritzers**: 10 to 100 percent of the total

- **Toners:** 50 to 100 percent of the total

- **Homemade creams and lotions:** Use for water portion of recipe

- **Cleansers:** approximately 1 teaspoon (5 ml) per ounce (28 ml) of liquid castile soap

To keep hydrosols fresh, it is important to keep them cool and away from direct light or heat. The average shelf life for most hydrosols is 12 to 24 months. Store hydrosols in a cool room or in the fridge to ensure freshness, stability, and liveliness of aroma. Stable, they can last up to 2 years.

Our Favorite Hydrosols

CALENDULA (*Calendula officinalis*): Calendula hydrosol is the best when it comes to having a first aid kit hydrosol, although using it with lavender or helichrysum hydrosols would make it even better. Prized for its wound healing, skin soothing, and antiseptic properties, calendula hydrosol can be used in gels or by itself for first aid. Spray on insect bites, mild cuts and scrapes, sunburns, and other inflamed skin conditions.

CLARY SAGE (*Salvia sclarea*): If ever there were a hydrosol for women of all ages, clary sage hydrosol would be it. Offering a powerful feminine energy, it can be spritzed into the air, used in a nourishing foot bath or full body bath, or sprayed on one's pillow after a long stressful day.

ROSE GERANIUM (*Pelargonium graveolens* var. *roseum*): Rose geranium hydrosol, like its essential oil, offers balance to the skin and the mind. Slightly astringent, rose geranium is indicated for oily skin conditions and can be beneficial as a toner for acne. The aroma calms and soothes the emotions.

GERMAN CHAMOMILE (*Matricaria chamomilla* (syn. *Matricaria recutita*)): German chamomile is an amazing hydrosol for cooling inflamed conditions, including emotional states such as irritability and anger. It's soothing for children and infants, whom it can help to fall asleep. Its ability to soothe inflamed skin conditions makes it a beneficial addition to a gel for applying to a sunburn.

HELICHRYSUM (*Helichrysum italicum*): Helichrysum is a wonderful hydrosol for wound healing, both physical and emotional. Aromatic sprays using helichrysum can be applied directly to a cut or burn to help keep the wound clean and to support the wound healing process. Helichrysum reduces inflammation and supports cellular regeneration.

LAVENDER (*Lavandula angustifolia*): Lavender, along with German chamomile, are our go-to hydrosols for infants and young children as well as the skin. Sprayed into the air, lavender hydrosol can calm emotions and prepare young ones for bed. It could also be used in a water-based diffusor to lightly scent the air for a good night's sleep. Lavender hydrosol can also be used in infant baths or as a linen spray.

NEROLI, also called orange flower (*Citrus aurantium* var. *amara*): beautiful and floral, slightly astringent, yet expansively compassionate and gentle, Neroli hydrosol is a great facial toner for oily skin types or for those who are being emotionally affected by the appearance, however transitional, of their skin. Neroli hydrosol's aroma is like a warm sunshine embrace.

ROSE (*Rosa × damascena*): Rose hydrosol is much loved for its beautiful aroma and gentleness to the heart and skin. It is a wonderful hydrosol for oily skin as well as for bug or insect bites, mild cuts and scrapes, and heat rash from the sun. Aromatically, rose hydrosol sprayed into the air can calm and soothe the heart, relieve tension, and nourish the mind.

WITCH HAZEL (*Hamamelis virginiana*): Witch hazel is often sold at pharmacy stores and is diluted down with rubbing alcohol. And although it is still used for cleaning wounds and supporting tissue healing, the hydrosol, in and of itself, is also used for bug or insect bites, mild cuts and scrapes, cleansing mild wounds, and reducing heat rash. Unlike other hydrosols, witch hazel hydrosol (without alcohol) has a shelf life of 8–12 months.

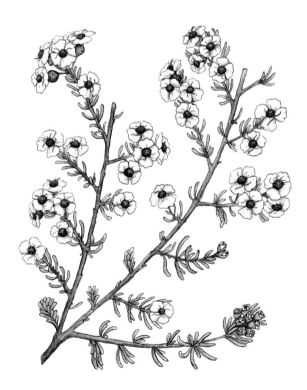

CHAPTER SEVEN

BODY CARE APPLICATIONS

PERHAPS THE MOST AMAZING THING about essential oils is that there are so many ways in which to use them. In this chapter, we will explore the most popular ways to integrate them into your life, wellness apothecary, and home. Let's begin our exploration with body and facial oils.

⇢ Body and Facial Oils

Making your own body or facial oil is a great way to enjoy the benefits of aroma while also supporting the health of your skin and body! Body oils not only nourish the skin, they are also beneficial for relieving stress, providing pain relief, and relieving muscle spasms or cramps. You can also relieve tension in the neck and upper back from sitting at a computer all day by applying an aromatic body oil to that area. Body oils can also be used for massage. If you are planning a visit to a massage therapist, consider asking them to use a massage oil you made yourself.

Facial oils, on the other hand, are specifically designed to nourish the facial skin. Facial oils will often contain special carrier oils such as rosehip seed oil, sea buckthorn, and calendula herbal oil.

WHAT YOU NEED
- Essential oils
- Carrier oil(s)
- Herbal oil(s)

- Antioxidant, if using rosehip seed or other omega-3 rich vegetable oils
- Bottle; use either a glass bottle with phenolic cap or a PET bottle

  ▷ For facial oils, we recommend making up 1 fluid ounce (30 ml) at a time

  ▷ For body oils, we recommend 2 to 4 fluid ounces (60 to 120 ml) at a time

- Glass measuring cup
- Blank label

Shelf Life: Six to twelve months from time the product is made. However, we recommend using handmade products up within a three- to six-month period. We believe that once blended into a carrier oil, the aromatics begin to slowly age. As they age, they begin to lose their vitality.

PROCEDURE

1. Decide how much oil you will be making.

2. Select one to three essential oils to be used for a blend.

3. Select carrier oil(s).

4. Measure your ingredients depending on the dilution:

   ▷ For body oils, you will need a total of 15 to 20 drops of essential oil per fluid ounce (30 ml).

   ▷ For facial oils, you will need a total of 7 to 14 drops per fluid ounce (30 ml).

5. Place all essential oil drops in the bottle. Swivel or shake the bottle.

6. Pour in carrier oil(s). Cap tightly and shake until well combined.

7. Name your oil blend and label the bottle with its name and ingredients. Be sure to put the date when the product was made!

⇀ Roll-On (aka Roller Balls)

We love these roll-on bottles! The roller ball is basically a 0.35 ounces (10 ml) bottle with a cap or lid that contains a ball. They're not only useful for application, they make great holiday gifts for your friends.

Each roller bottle holds 0.3 ounces (9 ml) of base oil. Choose what you have in stock: jojoba, sesame, rosehip seed, calendula herbal oil, or the like. Base oils add nourishment and may add color (e.g., unrefined avocado oil makes the oil a rich green color) and/or an aroma (e.g., raspberry seed oil gives it a raspberry-like aroma). The possibilities are endless.

The average number of drops of essential oils to use is between 5 to 12, depending on which are being used and the goal of your roller ball formulation. For example, you could use less of essential oils such as sandalwood or rose or more of monoterpene-rich essential oils, like the conifers or citrus essential oils.

PROCEDURE

It helps to have small beakers, such as in 1.75 ounces (50 ml) or 3.5 ounces (100 ml) sizes, on hand, but a small measuring cup works too.

1. Fill beaker with the carrier oil of your choice.

2. Pour oil into the bottle, just to the lip (where the side begins to turn in and go up). You don't want to fill it up to the very top!

3. Add in your drops of essential oil(s).

4. Holding a clean fingertip over the top, shake the bottle vigorously.

5. Smell the final blend to make sure it smells the way you would like it to. Adjust as necessary.

6. Place the ball and cap onto the inside lid.

7. Place the cap on the bottle.

8. Label the bottle. It's ready to be used.

TO MAKE A BATCH OF 10 AROMATHERAPY ROLLER BALLS

1. Measure out 3 fluid ounces (90 ml) of base oil(s).

2. Measure out 70 drops of essential oil synergy (see page 189) or a single essential oil.

3. Combine essential oil synergy with carrier oil.

4. Stir with a metal or glass stir rod until well combined.

5. Pour blend into each bottle, filling just to where the lip begins to turn up.

6. Pop ball/lids into bottles, then cap.

7. Place a label on each bottle.

8. Give to friends and family!

Roll-on Combinations

Compassion and Strength

- 0.3 ounce (9 ml) Jojoba oil
- 2 drops Neroli (*Citrus aurantium var. amara*) essential oil
- 3 drops Petitgrain (*Citrus aurantium var. amara*) essential oil
- 3 drops Tangerine (*Citrus reticulata*) essential oil

Forest Blend

- 0.3 ounce (9 ml) Jojoba oil
- 2 drops Pinyon Pine (*Pinus edulis*) essential oil
- 4 drops Scots Pine (*Pinus sylvestris*) essential oil
- 3 drops Cypress (*Cupressus sempervirens*) essential oil

Calm and Nourish

- 0.3 ounce (9 ml) Jojoba oil
- 2 drops Ylang Ylang (*Cananga odorata*) essential oil
- 1 to 2 drops Neroli (*Citrus aurantium var. amara*) essential oil
- 1 drop Cardamom (*Elettaria cardamomum*) essential oil
- 2 drops Sweet Orange (*Citrus sinensis*) essential oil

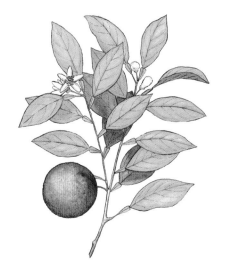

→ Body Butters

Body butters provide a nutrient-dense product to help heal and soothe damaged, weakened, or stressed skin. They have the remarkable capacity to heal tissue, soften dry areas of skin such as the elbows, knees, or feet, and perhaps most importantly, protect the skin's barrier function by preventing water loss. Body butters are most commonly used for dry, itchy skin conditions (where itchiness is caused by dryness) and to protect the skin from moisture loss, such as during the winter months when our skin is dealing with the cold and windy weather along with heat inside our living and working areas.

Body butters are made utilizing natural butters along with at least one carrier and/or herbal oil. Body butters do not contain water, so they do not need a preservative. However, depending on which vegetable oils you use in your formulation, you may want to consider adding in 1 percent antioxidant such as rosemary CO_2 extract, vitamin E, or mixed tocopherols.

WHAT YOU NEED
- A butter (e.g., shea butter) that is not cocoa; cocoa butter is not used to make body butters except when added in a low percentage to avoid making the butter too hard.
- Essential oils
- Carrier oil(s)
- Herbal oil(s)

Shelf Life:
- Most butters are good for up to 6 to 12 months.

- Depending on which base oils you choose, you may consider adding in 1 percent vitamin E or 0.5 percent to 1 percent rosemary CO_2 extract. We recommend adding one of these antioxidants to a body butter when using vegetable oils such as flax, rosehip seed, evening primrose, or borage.

Whipped Body Butter

A beautiful nourishing whipped body butter for the winter months.

Prep Time: 60 minutes
Yield: 8 ounces (225 g)

WHAT YOU NEED
- 8 ounces (225 g) shea butter
- 1 tablespoon (15 ml) Calendula herbal oil
- 12 drops Lavender (*Lavandula angustifolia*) essential oil
- 10 drops Tangerine (*Citrus reticulata*) essential oil
- 7 drops Petitgrain (*Citrus aurantium* var. *amara*) essential oil

PROCEDURE
1. Place the shea butter in a glass mixing bowl (taller than it is wide with this small amount) and begin whipping it with a hand-held mixer (on the whipping or high setting).

2. Once slightly whipped (it will still be somewhat "solid" and not as fluffy as the final product), add in Calendula herbal oil and the essential oils.

3. Continue to whip for 10 to 20 minutes. The longer the better!

4. Scoop it into an 8- or 16-ounce (250 or 500 ml) jar. Let the whipped butter stay "fluffy" in the jar!

5. Apply to the body as needed. Great to apply after a shower to help moisturize the skin and prevent dehydration.

➜ Aromatic Gels

Aromatic gels are used for insect bites, bruises, sunburns, small burns, and muscular aches and pains (e.g., shoulders and neck area), on the temples to soothe headaches, and to soothe inflamed or irritated skin. Gels are cooling by nature. The most commonly used gel for making aromatherapy products is aloe vera gel. Aloe vera gel has a long history of use in treating simple burns, including sunburn. Aloe vera gel may also be used to make homemade hand sanitizers.

Prep Time: 30 minutes
Yield: Varies
Shelf Life: Store gels in a cool room or fridge. Unpreserved gels or gels made with commercial aloe vera gel or gelly (which do have a basic preservative system) can last up to 1 to 3 months. With gels, it is a good idea to make up only a small amount, approximately 2 to 4 ounces (60 to 120 ml) at a time.

WHAT YOU NEED
- Essential oils
- Aloe vera gel or gelly
- Hydrosols

PROCEDURE
1. Select one to three essential oils.

2. Measure out a total of 10 to 15 drops of essential oil per ounce (30 ml) of aloe vera gel into a small bowl.

3. Measure aloe vera gel into the bowl.

4. Stir with a stainless-steel spoon or fork until well combined.

5. Scoop gel out of the bowl into a clean jar.

6. Label, being sure to list the ingredients.

7. Use as needed. Store in a cool area.

Natural Hand Protective Gel

Making your own hand gel, which soothes the skin while also protecting one from potential germs or infections, is empowering.

Prep Time: 5 minutes
Yield: 1 ounce (30 ml)

WHAT YOU NEED
- 1 fluid ounce (30 ml) aloe vera gel
- 7 drops Frankincense (*Boswellia sacra*) essential oil
- 3 drops Lavender (*Lavandula angustifolia*) essential oil
- 3 drops Myrrh (*Commiphora myrrha*) essential oil
- 7 drops Lemon (*Citrus limon*) essential oil

PROCEDURE
1. Combine all ingredients in a small bowl.

2. Pour into a 1-ounce (30 ml) PET bottle with a flip top.

3. Use as needed or desired throughout the day.

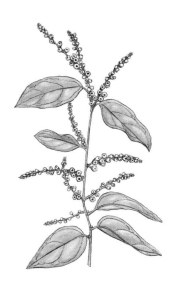

⇀ Salves

If you have ever used Vicks VapoRub, then you have used a type of salve. Aromatic salves are made up of beeswax, vegetable and/or herbal oils (e.g., Calendula), and essential oils. You can make salves thicker by simply adding more beeswax or semisolid by adding less beeswax. It's up to you!

Why use a salve? Salves are amazing for congestion and for small localized applications for such things as insect bites and dry patches of skin.

Prep Time: 60 minutes
Yield: Two 1 ounce (30 ml) jars and one 0.5 ounce (15 ml) jar
Safety: Salves should not be applied to poison ivy rashes, weepy eczema, pimples, boils, fresh sunburn, or fungal or bacterial skin infections.

WHAT YOU NEED
- Double boiler (stainless steel)
- Glass measuring cup
- Small scale to weigh beeswax
- Tins or glass jars
- Stainless steel fork or stirring rod
- Paper towels

INGREDIENTS
- ¼ cup (60 ml) vegetable and/or herbal oil/s
- ¼ ounce (7 g) beeswax or candelilla wax
- 30 to 50 drops essential oils

PROCEDURE
1. Clean the space where you will be making salve.

2. Clean all utensils, the double boiler, and the bowls or measuring cups.

3. Fill the bottom pot of the double boiler with 2 to 3 cups (500 to 700 ml) of water. Place the top pan on the bottom pot. Place the double boiler onto medium heat and heat water to just below boiling.

4. Add in wax. Allow it to begin melting, then add the carrier oils.

5. Stir ingredients together until well combined.

6. Once all the beeswax is melted, remove from heat and add in the essential oils.

7. Stir the essential oils quickly into the salve mixture.

8. Pour salve into jars or tins. If the salve begins to harden, place the pot back onto the double boiler (turn heat back on if necessary).

9. Place a cap on the jars or tins and allow the salve to harden.

10. Check salves to make sure you like the texture and that the aroma is of a desired strength based upon the goals of the salve.

11. Create labels for your salve jars and include all the ingredients.

12. Once salves are labeled, they are ready to use!

NOTE: Test the consistency of a salve before blending it with other essential oils by placing a spoonful of the salve in the refrigerator. Allow it to harden. If the salve comes out too hard or thick, you can melt the mixture down again and add more oil. If the salve is too fluid or thin, you can melt it down and mix in some more beeswax.

Dilution/dosage recommendation: The salve-making dosage may seem a bit high, but this is because a salve holds essential oils differently than other delivery systems do. Our recommended dosage is 30 to 40 drops per ounce (30 g) of salve.

⇢ Lip Balms

Lip balms are fun and easy to make using simple ingredients. The recipe provided below is our all-time favorite formulation much loved by all who use it.

Yield: 10 to 15 lip balm tubes
Prep Time: 15 minutes

INGREDIENTS
- 20 g beeswax
- 1.4 ounces (40 g) vanilla-infused jojoba oil (available to purchase from a variety of aromatherapy companies) or use regular jojoba oil or other vegetable oil of choice
- 25 g shea butter
- 15 g cocoa butter

WHAT YOU NEED
- 10 to15 lip balm tubes or other acceptable containers
- Two to three 1 to 2 ounces (30-50 ml) salve jars (for the lips and body)
- Stainless steel double boiler
- Scale that weighs in grams
- Stainless steel fork (for stirring)
- Paper towels
- Optional: tray that holds lip balm tubes steady

PROCEDURE
1. Weigh all ingredients carefully.

2. Prepare the double boiler by adding water to the bottom pot then place the top pot above it. Allow the water to come to a slow boil. Place beeswax in the top pot and allow it to melt.

3. Just as the beeswax is almost melted, add the vanilla-infused jojoba and shea butter. Gently melt them down. Just before the shea butter is completely melted, add in cocoa butter (this will melt very quickly). Be sure to stir well!

4. Fill the containers. You can use a lip balm tray to help fill them if you have one.

5. Let the balms sit to harden. Wipe off the outside of the tubes or gently clean the jar lips with a paper towel.

Alternative to Beeswax: Candelilla Lip Balm

For this recipe, use the above instructions with the following adjustment in ingredients.

Yield: 12 lip balm tubes (0.15 ounces or 4.5 g each), plus a little extra

INGREDIENTS
- 2 tablespoons (30 g) candelilla wax
- 0.55 ounce or the equivalent of 7 cocoa butter chips (approximately 1½ tablespoons or 15 g)
- 2 tablespoons (30 g) shea butter
- 6 tablespoons (90 ml) vanilla jojoba oil
- 6 to 10 drops essential oils (e.g., peppermint, lavender, lime)

⤚ Salt Scrubs

We love salt scrubs. They stimulate circulation and remove dead skin cells while leaving the skin radiant. In creating a salt scrub, it is best to use a fine- to medium-sized sea salt. Epsom salt does not seem to work as well. Stay away from anything too coarse, as you don't want to scratch or damage the skin.

Prep Time: 15 to 30 minutes
Yield: This recipe will fill an 8-ounce (250 ml) jar.
Safety: Never apply salt scrub to broken skin. Salt can irritate the skin if used right after shaving or waxing. It's best to avoid salt scrubs for 24 to 48 hours after you do either.

WHAT YOU NEED

- 2 cups (540 g) sea salt
- ½ cup (120 ml) natural vegetable oil such as almond, apricot, or sunflower
- 7 to 25 drops essential oil(s), depending on the usage and strength desired

PROCEDURE

1. In a small bowl, mix sea salt and vegetable oil.

2. Add essential oils.

3. Stir until well combined.

TO USE:

1. Wet the skin, either in the shower (then turn off the water) or by using a hydrosol or aromatic spritzer.

2. Apply the salt glow treatment to the desired area. Use quick, vigorous strokes or make it more relaxing with longer, slower strokes. The important thing is to keep the mixture and circulation moving.

3. Remove or rinse the mixture from the body by taking a warm shower.

4. Avoid using salt scrubs on the face, as this skin is too delicate and prone to scratching.

5. Be sure to conclude your salt glow with a natural moisturizing oil or lotion to feed and replenish the newly exfoliated skin.

Variations on the traditional salt glow can be achieved by incorporating dried herbs, ground nuts, seaweeds, and other natural ingredients.

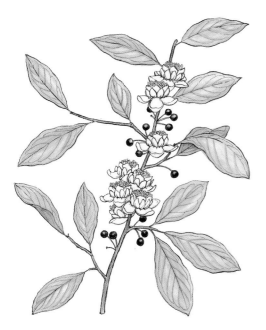

⇸ Aromatic Baths

Bathing is a wonderful way to enjoy the beauty of the aromas of essential oils while relaxing in warm water. Bathing with essential oils can reduce stress, emotional tension, and anxiety, and it can relieve muscular tension. Have trouble sleeping? Consider taking an evening aromatic bath with essential oils by candlelight.

Prep Time: 5 to 15 minutes
Yield: 1 bath
Safety: Avoid placing essential oils into the bath prior to getting into the bath. Do not use skin-irritating essential oils such as thyme, oregano, lemongrass, cinnamon bark or leaf, or other phenol- or aldehyde-rich essential oils in the bath. Avoid using extra drops of essential oil. A few drops go a long way. Be cautious when using citrus or conifer essential oils. We recommend 2 to 3 drops for these essential oils.

WHAT YOU NEED

- Essential oil(s)
- Honey, liquid castile soap, solubol, glycerin, full-fat milk, vegetable oil, herbal oil, or another "dispersing" agent
- Small glass bowl (to blend in)

PROCEDURE

1. Add 3 to 7 drops of essential oil(s) into 1 table-spoon (30 ml) honey.

2. Once in the bath, gently pour the mixture into the bathwater. Use your fingers to remove any remaining product from the bowl.

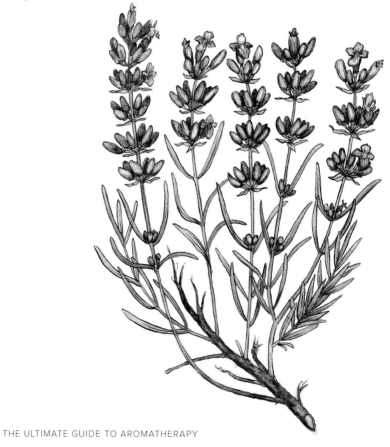

⇀ Body and Facial Cleansers

Cleaning the skin is one of the most common rituals we have as humans. Who doesn't love to take a nice warm shower, either at the beginning or end of the day? The ritual of cleansing seems to provide one with a sense of rejuvenation. Body and facial cleansers are designed to remove dead skin cells, grime, excess sebum, stale makeup, sweat, and bacteria from the skin.

The most common cleanser used to make aromatherapy cleansers is liquid castile soap, an all-natural, vegetable-based cleansing product.

Prep Time: 15 to 30 minutes
Yield: Varies
Shelf Life: 6 to 12 months. However, we recommend using handmade products up within a 3- to 6-month period. We believe that once blended into a base, the aromatics will slowly begin to age and lose their vitality.

WHAT YOU NEED
- Essential oil(s)
- Unscented liquid castile soap (often available at a local natural health or grocery store). We recommend Dr. Bronner's Baby Unscented Pure-Castile Liquid Soap

PROCEDURE
1. Select one to three essential oils.
2. Add a total of 10 to 15 drops of essential oil per ounce (28 ml) of liquid castile soap.
3. Combine ingredients in a PET or glass bottle.

Aromatherapy Foaming Cleanser for Hands

Here's how to make your own aromatic foaming cleanser.

WHAT YOU NEED
- Organic liquid castile soap
- Hydrosol of choice (German chamomile or lavender works well)
- Essential oil(s) of choice
- Organic aloe vera gel
- Organic vegetable glycerin
- Whisk
- Measuring cup
- PET container with a foamer pump

INGREDIENTS
- ¾ cup (175 ml) castile soap
- ¼ cup (60 ml) German chamomile hydrosol
- 1 tablespoon (15 ml) organic vegetable glycerin
- 2 tablespoons (30 ml) aloe vera gel
- 25 drops lavender essential oil
- 20 drops tea tree or eucalyptus radiata essential oil

PROCEDURE
1. Place castile soap into a glass measuring cup.
2. Add organic vegetable glycerin, aloe vera gel, and German chamomile hydrosol.
3. Add essential oil(s).
4. Gently whisk all ingredients together.
5. Pour mixture into a cleanser bottle and cap with a foamer top.
6. Label the bottle with the ingredients. Cleansing soap is now ready to use.

⤙ Creams and Lotions

Ever have dry skin? It's quite common, and it becomes even more common as we age due to changes in the skin. Other contributing factors to dry skin include lack of water and healthy fats in the diet. Make sure to cultivate a healthy diet that includes healthy fats and ensure you have a good water intake throughout the day.

When it comes to aromatherapy and dry skin, creams and lotions are your best tools. They offer both oil and water to soften and soothe skin while supporting its ability to retain moisture. What's the difference between a cream and a lotion? Creams tend to be thicker than lotions and are commonly used on the face or on localized dry spots on the body. Lotions, on the other hand, tend to be thinner in texture and can be applied to the whole body.

The easiest way to incorporate essential oils into creams and lotions is to start with a cream or lotion on the market that you like and that works for your skin.

Prep Time: 15 to 30 minutes
Yield: Varies
Shelf Life: Most unscented creams and lotions commonly available in health food stores will have some type of preservative system. We recommend using cream or lotion up within 6 to 12 months. If using an unpreserved cream or lotion, the shelf life tends to be 1 to 6 months depending on how it is stored and used.

WHAT YOU NEED
- Unscented cream or lotion
- Essential oil(s)
- Bowl
- Spoon
- Silicone spatula

PROCEDURE
1. Select 3 to 5 essential oils (use an equal number of drops of each for the total number of recommended drops).

2. Measure and place the cream or lotion in a clean bowl.

3. Add in appropriate drops of each essential oil:
   ▷ Cream for face: 4 to 6 drops per ounce (30 ml); or
   ▷ Lotion: 7 to 14 drops per ounce (30 ml).

4. Stir the essential oil(s) into the cream or lotion using a stainless steel spoon. Stir until well combined.

5. Scoop the cream or lotion into a clean container.

6. Name the product, create a label, and place the label on the jar. Be sure to list all the ingredients so you know what's in it.

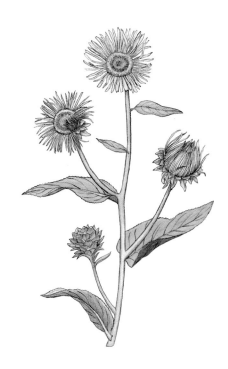

CHAPTER EIGHT

DIFFUSION AND INHALATION

Diffusing essential oils into the air or inhaling them is a great way to relieve stress and anxiety, support a good night's rest, increase alertness, improve air quality, and reduce airborne germs. While diffusion of essential oils tends to affect everyone within the environment being diffused, inhalation tends to be a personal interaction with the essential oils. With both diffusion and inhalation, you will be making a synergy of essential oils. A **synergy** is a combination of essential oils without a carrier/herbal oil or other base (e.g., cream, lotion, or gel). Synergies are designed to be used in diffusers (all types), in personal inhalers, or for steam inhalations.

You can also use hydrosols in some of the methods of application for diffusion and inhalation. See the chart below.

DIFFUSION

The most common tools used to diffuse essential oils into the environment are:

1. WATER DIFFUSER, ALSO KNOWN AS AN ULTRA-SONIC DIFFUSER. This type of diffuser uses an internal diaphragm that vibrates at an ultrasonic frequency, which involves sound waves with a frequency above the upper limit of human hearing. This ultrasonic vibration turns the water into vapor, which carries essential oil molecules (aroma) into the atmosphere. These are great diffusers for smaller spaces in the home, such as a bedroom, home office, or living room. They are simple to use. Typically, add water to the bowl and add 5 to 10 drops of essential oil or synergy. Allow the diffusor to run for 15 to 30 minutes every hour.

2. CANDLE DIFFUSER. Candle diffusors are a great way to benefit mood, energy, and other emotional states. Typically, candle diffusers are a piece of pottery designed with a small bowl on top and a place for a tealight candle underneath the bowl. The tealight gently warms the water in the bowl, which contains drops of an essential oil or a synergy of essential oils. The heating of the water slowly diffuses the aroma of the essential oil(s) into the environment.

This is a beautiful way to enjoy the aroma of the essential oil(s) along with the ambience of a tealight, and it is simple to use. Fill the bowl with water and add 5 to 10 drops of an essential oil or synergy. Light the candle and place it underneath the bowl. Add more essential oil if needed. Allow the diffuser to go until the water is almost gone.

Safety:
- Do not leave a candle diffuser unattended.
- Keep a lit candle out of the reach of children.

- **Clean regularly** with hot soapy water. Dry the unit, and then wipe with a paper towel and a bit of rubbing alcohol. You don't want mold growing in there!

3. NEBULIZING DIFFUSER. This is an electric diffuser typically made out of three pieces: the base (a kind of pump that will blow air into the glass "nebulizer"), the glass nebulizer, and a small piece of glass that is placed onto the nebulizer to direct microdroplets of essential oil into the atmosphere. These microdroplets are suspended in the air for a short while.

This type of diffuser tends to be used in more clinical settings or by aromatherapy practitioners, although it can certainly be used in the home as well. The nebulizing diffuser is often the most expensive option for diffusing essential oils into the environment.

To clean the diffuser, soak the glass part in a solution of 70 percent alcohol or 100 percent rubbing alcohol or even vodka, for a few hours. Rinse with hot water and allow to dry completely before the next use.

Usage and Safety:

- **Nebulizing diffusers are designed to be used 10 to 15 minutes every hour or 30 minutes every two hours. Do not run them continuously!** We were once told a story about this by the director of the integrative health services at the now-closed San Diego Hospice. During their research on the impact of essential oils being diffused via a nebulizer into a patient's room, she observed that when the diffuser was left on too long, the patient often began responding to the aromatics in the opposite direction. When it was on for 10 to 15 minutes, the patient would be relaxed and soothed. When it was left on for too long, the patient would become agitated. Lesson learned. Too much of anything is not a good thing!

- **Avoid the use of viscous essential oils** such as vetiver or sandalwood, as these oils may clog the unit and can get a bit gummy, making them difficult (though not impossible) to remove. Use the cleaning method described above and soak it for a longer time. We have also found that using lemongrass essential oil can be beneficial in removing gummy stuff from glassware.

- **Avoid using expensive essential oils** such as melissa or rose. There are other less expensive essential oils with similar properties to diffuse.

- **Do not use vegetable or other carrier oils** in a nebulizing diffuser.

INHALATION/DIFFUSION		
	SY	HY
DIFFUSION		
Ultrasonic (water) diffuser	X	X
Candle diffuser	X	X
Nebulizing diffuser	X	
Aromatic spritzer	X	X
Personal inhaler	X	
Steam inhalation	X	X

Key to codes:

SY Synergy: a combination of 3–5 essential oils without a base/carrier oil

HY Hydrosol(s): also known as hydrolats, are one of the products of the distillation process

⇻ Aromatic Spritzers

Aromatic spritzers, also known as room sprays or linen sprays, have become popular for their ability not only to freshen and cleanse the air but also to uplift, relax, or energize those who are exposed to their aromas. Aromatic spritzers can also be used to reduce yucky odors in the air or to "scent" clothing, bed linens, and fabric on furniture.

The basic ingredients of aromatic spritzers are water (can use hydrosols 100 percent) and essential oils. We recommend using distilled water when possible and affordable. If not, tap water is fine too. For home use, water is fine, but you could also use vodka as the base for the spritzer. Or if you happen to have 190 proof grain alcohol hanging around, you could dilute it with water to 70 percent and use this as your base. The benefit of using 70 percent alcohol is that essential oils are soluble into the alcohol and no emulsifier would be needed. What is an emulsifier? An emulsifier is something that helps disperse essential oils into the water and reduces the need to shake the product with each use. Although beneficial if you're making a product line for retail sale, this is really unnecessary for home use and only adds to the cost of spritzer.

Yield: Depends on the size of the bottle (2 to 8 ounces (60 to 240 ml) is what we recommend)
Prep Time: 30 minutes
Shelf Life: If made with distilled water only, 1 to 3 months when stored in a cool place. If made with 70 percent alcohol (and 30 percent water), store 6 to 12 months. We recommend using aromatic spritzers within 6 months if possible. This ensures the vitality of the aroma.

WHAT YOU NEED

- Spritzer bottle: We recommend a 2 to 8 ounce (60 to 240 ml) round glass or PET bottle with a spritzer top
- Distilled water (available at grocery stores) or hydrosols
- Optional: vodka or 190 proof alcohol diluted down to 70 percent alcohol/30 percent water
- Optional: emulsifier such as Solubol

PROCEDURE

1. Select one to three different, complementary essential oils, or a premade synergy.

2. Add a total of 10 to 15 drops of essential oil per ounce (30 ml) of water in a spritzer bottle. If using more than one essential oil, use equal drops of each to add up to 10 to 15 total drops.

3. Swivel the bottle to combine the oils.

4. Add distilled water or other chosen liquid.

5. Shake well prior to each use.

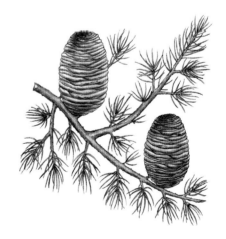

→ Personal Inhaler Tubes

Personal inhaler tubes can be used to relieve stress, uplift mood, reduce or relieve nausea (e.g., travel nausea), support emotional well-being, reduce sinus congestion, and provide support during challenging times.

Inhaler tubes are designed using 100 percent essential oil(s) saturated on a cotton pad. A personal inhaler is a fun and easy product to make and a safe method of application, so you can enjoy your inhaler throughout the day.

Prep Time: 15 to 30 minutes
Yield: 1 inhaler tube
Shelf Life: 6 to 12 months

WHAT YOU NEED
- Essential oils
- Small glass bowl
- Spoon
- Empty inhaler tube, including tube, cap, and cotton pad

PROCEDURE
1. Select two to three essential oils.

2. Decide how many drops of essential oil to use. We recommend a total of 20 to 25 drops to saturate the cotton pad. Equally divide drops among your chosen essential oils.

3. Add drops to a bowl.

4. Drop the cotton pad into the bowl and, using the tip of the spoon, gently move the pad around to soak up the oil.

5. Pick up the pad with tweezers or your fingers and insert it into the inhaler tube.

6. Place the bottom onto the inhaler tube and lid onto the top of the tube.

7. Be sure to create a label for the inhaler with ingredients listed.

8. Create a name for the inhaler based upon its purpose or therapeutic goal (e.g., Relax Inhaler).

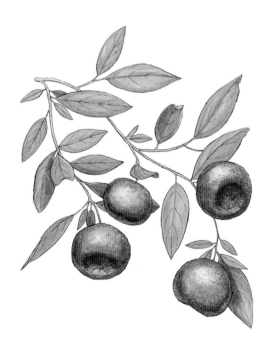

⇥ Smelling Salts

Making your own smelling salts is a great alternative to using the plastic personal inhalers. With growing concerns about the widespread use of plastic along with the challenges of disposing of it, we recommend you consider this as a wonderful way to enjoy the aromatic benefits of essential oils.

Prep Time: 10 to 20 minutes
Yield: 1 container of smelling salts
Shelf life: 6 to 12 months

WHAT YOU NEED
- Essential oils
- Fine- or medium-grind sea salt or Epsom salt
- ⅓ ounce (10 ml) European dropper bottle or other suitable small lidded glass container

PROCEDURE
1. Create a synergy with a total of 20 to 30 drops utilizing three to five essential oils. Place it in the glass container.

2. Gently shake the bottle to combine the oils.

3. Pour salt into the bottle.

4. Place the lid on the bottle and shake vigorously to coat all the salt with the synergy of essential oils.

5. Create a label for the bottle with its ingredients.

6. Name the salts based on their purpose or therapeutic goal.

⇥ Inhaler to Relieve Emotional Turmoil from PMS

AUTHOR: Amandine Peter

Geranium helps relieve stress and anxiety while balancing hormones, ylang ylang provides a sense of euphory and well-being, and patchouli and bergamot relieve the depression and irritation associated with premenstrual syndrome.

Prep Time: 10 to 15 minutes
Makes: 1 inhaler
Safety: No concerns

INGREDIENTS
- 4 drops Rose Geranium (*Pelargonium graveolens* var. *roseum*) essential oil
- 4 drops Ylang Ylang (*Cananga odorata*) essential oil
- 7 drops Patchouli (*Pogostemon cablin*) essential oil
- 10 drops Bergamot (*Citrus bergamia*) essential oil

ALTERNATIVE ESSENTIAL OILS:
For Geranium: Clary Sage (*Salvia sclarea*) or Lavender (*Lavandula angustifolia*)
For Ylang Ylang: Roman Chamomile (*Chamaemelum nobile*), Neroli (*Citrus aurantium* var. *amara*), or Petitgrain (*Citrus aurantium* var. *amara*)
For Patchouli: Frankincense (*Boswellia sacra*) or Vetiver (*Chrysopogon (Vetiveria) zizanioides*)
For Bergamot: Sweet Orange (*Citrus sinensis*) or Red Mandarin (*Citrus reticulata*)

→ Steam Inhalation

When Amandine Peter, one of the senior instructors at our school, was a child, her mother would boil up some water and then pour it into a bowl on the kitchen table for Amy and her sisters to do steam inhalations when they were congested or had a cold. Amy loved putting the towel over her head and breathing in the warm vapors of steam and a bit of Vicks VapoRub.

Steam inhalations are incredibly beneficial for loosening congestion in the nasal cavity, allowing mucus to be thinned and expelled by blowing the nose. Steam inhalations with essential oils may also be used for things such as sinusitis, to help relieve inflammation and open up the nasal passages.

Steam inhalation is one of the most effective methods of application when it comes to affections of the respiratory system. The steam carries active compounds from the essential oils directly into the nose and down to the lungs. It is also easy to prepare. The following recipe just requires water and essential oils.

Prep time: 15 minutes
Yield: 1 steam inhalation treatment
Safety: Avoid irritating essential oils such as oregano, thyme ct. thymol, cinnamon bark or cinnamon leaf. Be cautious using peppermint essential oil. Use only 1 drop. Do not open your eyes while doing steam inhalation. Avoid steam inhalations for children under the age of 5 years.

WHAT YOU NEED

- 1 to 3 essential oils
- 4 cups (950 ml) water
- Cooking pot or kettle
- Bowl for hot water
- Towel

SOME ESSENTIAL OILS TO CONSIDER INCLUDE:

Eucalyptus (either *Eucalyptus globulus* or *Eucalyptus radiata*), Thyme ct. linalool (*Thymus vulgaris*), Lemon (*Citrus limon*), Green Myrtle (*Myrtus communis*)

PROCEDURE

1. Select one to three essential oil(s).

2. Place water in a pot or kettle and bring it to a boil.

3. Pour boiling water into the bowl.

4. Prepare to do inhalations by placing the towel around your shoulders.

5. Place 1 to 2 drops of each essential oil into the bowl. The total should equal between 3 and 5 drops.

6. Place the towel over your head, shut your eyes, and bend over the steam. Take 5 to 10 deep slow breaths in through the nose.

7. Once complete, if water is still hot, you can repeat steps 5 and 6.

Steam Inhalation for Bronchitis

AUTHOR: Amandine Peter

While eucalyptus and niaouli possess strong anti-bacterial, antiviral, and expectorant effects, lemon is known for enhancing the immune system, and inula helps break down mucus with an added anti-inflammatory benefit.

This inhalation can be used two to three times a day.

Yield: 1 inhalation
Prep Time: 10 to 20 minutes
Safety: Eucalyptus and Niaouli ct. cineole should be avoided by children via this route

WHAT YOU NEED

- 2 cups (475 ml) water
- 1 drop Eucalyptus (*Eucalyptus globulus*) essential oil
- 1 drop Niaouli ct. cineole (*Melaleuca quinquenervia*) essential oil
- 1 drop Lemon (*Citrus limon*) essential oil
- 1 drop Inula (*Dittrichia graveolens* syn. *Inula graveolens*) essential oil

ALTERNATIVE ESSENTIAL OILS:

For Eucalyptus: Eucalyptus radiata (*Eucalyptus radiata*) or Rosemary ct. cineole (*Rosmarinus officinalis*)
For Niaouli: Tea Tree (*Melaleuca alternifolia*) or Laurel (*Laurus nobilis*)
For Lemon: Frankincense (*Boswellia sacra*) or Scots Pine (*Pinus sylvestris*)
For Inula: Helichrysum (*Helichrysum italicum*) or Lavender (*Lavandula angustifolia*)

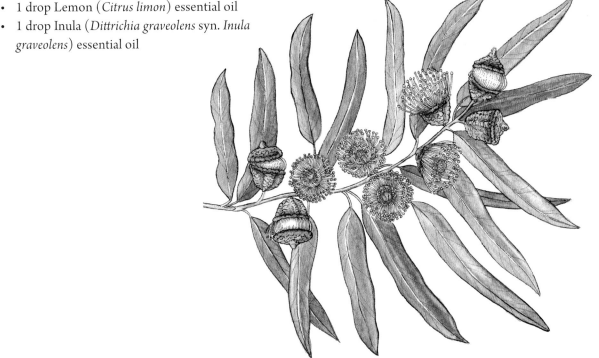

PART V

Putting It All Together

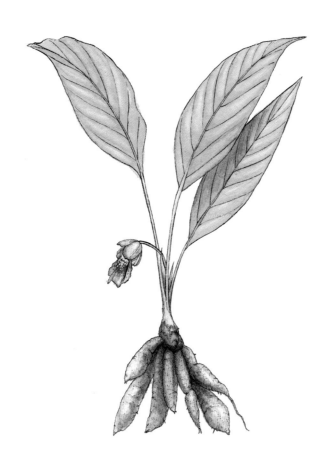

CHAPTER NINE

AROMATIC REMEDIES

THIS CHAPTER features several remedies to reach for when they're needed. See page 10 for more on using aromatherapy to improve health and well-being.

⇢ Salve for Joint Pain

AUTHOR: Amy Anthony

Cold, dull joint pain could discourage anyone from getting on the move! It may also affect the surrounding muscles needed to support mobility, making them tired and sore. Ginger, sweet basil, and clove offer pain relief while bringing blood and heat to the treated area. Copaiba and Lavendin further support pain relief and bring in powerful anti-inflammatory properties. Arnica-infused oil brings further pain relief. Sesame is warming and deeply penetrating, helping the essential oils go deep into tissues.

INGREDIENTS

- 20 drops Lavender (*Lavandula angustifolia*) essential oil
- 20 drops Copaiba (*Copaifera officinalis*) essential oil
- 10 drops Ginger (*Zingiber officinale*) essential oil
- 10 drops Sweet Basil ct. linalool (*Ocimum basilicum*) essential oil
- 5 drops Clove (*Syzygium aromaticum*) essential oil
- 1 tablespoon (15 g) Beeswax
- 2 tablespoons (30 ml) Arnica (*Arnica montana*) herbal oil
- 1½ tablespoons (22 ml) Sesame oil

Yield: Approximately 2 ounces (50 g)
Prep Time: 20 minutes
Safety: Do not use arnica herbal oil on open wounds or cuts. This product is designed for those 14 years of age or older.

WHAT YOU NEED

- Heatproof measuring cups or beakers
- Measuring spoons
- Double boiler
- Glass, stainless steel, or wooden stirrer
- 2-ounce (50 ml) glass or metal jar with cap
- Label

1. Place about 1 inch (2.5 cm) of water in the bottom pot of the double boiler and place it over medium heat.

2. Place the second pot on top of it to create your double boiler (you may choose to put a small amount of water (½ inch or 1 cm) in this pot as well).

3. Place a heatproof measuring cup into the second pot. Place the beeswax in the measuring cup and allow it to melt.

4. Slowly add the arnica and sesame oil to the wax and stir to incorporate it.

5. Take the glass measuring cup out of the double boiler and wipe it off to ensure no water gets into the salve or the salve container.

6. Drop the essential oils directly into the beeswax and arnica/sesame oil mixture.

7. Stir well to incorporate.

8. Transfer the salve to the glass or tin jar and immediately affix the cap.

9. Label the salve and set aside for 24 hours to set.

How to Use Salve for Joint Pain: Apply a generous amount of salve to pain sites. Gently massage the salve into the pain site. Use as needed. Use within 6 months.

NOTE: If you do not have access to an arnica-infused oil, you can substitute another kind of oil such as sesame or sunflower. Arnica was chosen for its additional pain-relieving qualities. Sesame has antioxidants and a deeply penetrating nature, allowing essential oils to go deep into tissues.

ALTERNATE ESSENTIAL OILS:
Black Pepper (*Piper nigrum*), Scots Pine (*Pinus sylvestris*), and Rosemary (*Rosmarinus officinalis*)

NOTE: This is blended at a 5 percent dilution, which is highlighted for use in salves. That means 60 drops of essential oil in a 2-ounce (50 g) product.

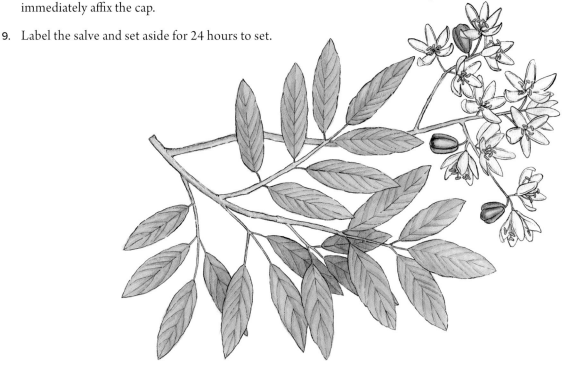

→ Tummy Massage Oil to Help Prevent Indigestion

AUTHOR: Elisabeth Vlasic

Dyspepsia is a common complaint in today's fast-paced world. It affects the upper gastrointestinal organs—small intestine, stomach, and esophagus—and can be caused by underlying emotional issues (stress), eating too much food, eating too fast, eating spicy foods, eating unsuitable food combinations, and the activity of pathogens and even food allergies. Indigestion can cause a broad range of unpleasant responses in the body including flatulence, bloating, heartburn, tummy pain, and nausea.

Essential oils with settling and soothing attributes can subside the effects of dyspepsia by working to stimulate digestion and relaxing digestive muscles, thus restoring balance. If digestive upset is triggered by pathogens, the essential oils can eliminate them, creating a healthier environment.

This massage oil is best used as a preventive measure to prelude digestion, but it can also be used in between meals or after eating if preferred.

Prep Time: 25 minutes
Yield: Approximately 1 ounce (30 ml)
Safety: Not a suitable remedy for children. Marjoram should be avoided with asthma.

INGREDIENTS

- 7 drops Fingerroot (*Boesenbergia rotunda*) essential oil
- 7 drops Cardamom (*Elettaria cardamomum*) essential oil
- 7 drops Ginger (*Zingiber officinale*) essential oil
- 5 drops Sweet Marjoram (*Origanum majorana*) essential oil
- 4 drops Cilantro (*Coriandrum sativum*) essential oil
- 1 ounce (28 ml) Jojoba oil (*Simmondsia chinensis*)

WHAT YOU NEED

- 1 small glass beaker or stainless steel or glass bowl
- Glass, stainless steel, or wooden stirrer or spoon
- 1-ounce (30 ml) glass bottle with dropper lid
- Small funnel
- Label

PROCEDURE

1. Place fingerroot, cardamom, ginger, marjoram and cilantro essential oils directly into the 1-ounce (30 ml) glass bottle.

2. Gently swirl the bottle, ensuring the essential oils mix together well.

3. Cap tightly and label.

4. Store in a dark, cool place and use as needed.

How to Use Tummy Massage Oil to Relieve Indigestion: Apply Tummy Massage Oil to Help Prevent Indigestion for a few minutes in a clockwise motion before meals. This will help one's mind-body to prepare for "rest and digest," offering another way to help ease the digestion process besides the powerful effect of the essential oils.

ALTERNATE ESSENTIAL OILS: Carrot Seed (*Daucus carota* subsp. *carota*), Fennel (*Foeniculum vulgare*), and Sweet Orange (*Citrus sinensis*)

NOTE: Lavender (*Lavandula angustifolia*) and Cardamom (*Elettaria cardamomum*) are indicated for use with digestive concerns relating to emotional issues. This is determined at a 5 percent blend for general massage work. It works out to 30 drops of essential oils in a 1-ounce (30 ml) remedy.

⤳ Inhaler to Relieve Indigestion

AUTHOR: Amy Anthony

Indigestion woes! Heartburn may be caused by several things, such as rich fatty foods or eating too quickly, but an underlying cause may often be a sluggish liver and underactive gall bladder. Help get things moving by welcoming some spice-based essential oils into your routine. Ginger, fennel, and sweet orange all have an affinity for stimulating gastric juices and helping the body release excess gas, thus settling the digestive tract and helping you get on your way.

Prep Time: 5 minutes
Yield: 1 inhaler tube
Safety: Fennel seed essential oil should be avoided (any route of application) during pregnancy and breastfeeding and with children under 5 years, due to its trans-anethole content. It should also be avoided by those living with endometriosis and estrogen-dependent cancers.

INGREDIENTS
- 17 drops Sweet Orange (*Citrus sinensis*) essential oil
- 5 drops Fennel (*Foeniculum vulgare*) essential oil
- 3 drops Ginger (*Zingiber officinale*) essential oil

WHAT YOU NEED
- Inhaler tube with inhaler core
- Small glass or ceramic bowl
- Tweezers
- Label

PROCEDURE
1. Place essential oils into the bowl.

2. Swirl the bowl to combine them.

3. Place the inhaler core into the bowl, allowing it to absorb the essential oils until it is saturated. Help this along by using the tweezers to move around the inhaler core.

4. Place the saturated core into the inhaler tube using the tweezers.

5. Affix the bottom cap onto the tube. Ensure the inhaler cap is firmly screwed onto the inhaler and label.

How to Use Inhaler to Relieve Indigestion: You can use the inhaler after meals to relieve upset, but it is best to use it *before* meals to stimulate the digestive process and stave off discomfort.

Remove the cap and hold the Inhaler to Relieve Indigestion 1 inch (2.5 cm) from your nose, inhaling deeply for a few breaths. Keep the cap tightly on the inhaler when not in use to prevent essential oils from evaporating. Use within 3 months, as the essential oils evaporate over the use of the product.

ALTERNATE ESSENTIAL OILS: Cardamom (*Elettaria cardamomum*), Mandarin (*Citrus reticulata*), and Spearmint (*Mentha spicata*)

NOTE: Most inhaler blanks hold 25 to 30 drops of essential oil. Feel free to adjust the number of drops to the type of core you use. You may choose to forgo the typical inhaler core in favor of a square or circular organic cotton cosmetic pad; simply cut down to size for the tube.

↪ Soothing Bath Blend for Restless Legs: Stock Bottle

AUTHOR: Amy Anthony

Although the exact cause of Restless Leg Syndrome (RLS) continues to be sought, some relief may be realized by working with essential oils with known nervine-sedative activity. As RLS often gets worse at the end of the day, especially when trying to go to sleep, balancing and sedating essential oils such as petitgrain, palmarosa, and pinyon pine may be used in a calming bath and diffused before bed to calm the nervous system and promote a restful sleep.

Prep Time: 5 minutes
Yield: Approximately 24 baths

INGREDIENTS

- 60 drops Petitgrain (*Citrus aurantium* var. *amara*) essential oil
- 36 drops Palmarosa (*Cymbopogon martinii*) essential oil
- 24 drops Pinyon Pine (*Pinus edulis*) essential oil

WHAT YOU NEED

- 5 milliliter stock bottle with orifice reducer
- Label

PROCEDURE

1. Place essential oils into the 5 milliliter bottle.

2. Affix the cap and label.

How to Use Soothing Bath Blend for Restless Legs: Try adding a few drops of the Soothing Bath Blend for Restless Legs to a warm bath or diffuse in the bedroom 30 minutes before going to sleep.

To Incorporate the Synergy into a Bath: Draw a bath where the water is 100°F to 110°F (38°C to 43°C). Ensure there is enough water in the tub so a full-body immersion is possible. The water should be up to your neck and covering your heart. Add 1 to 2 cups (200 to 400 g) Magnesium Chloride or Magnesium Sulfate and 1 to 2 cups (200 to 400 g) Dead Sea Salt to the bath. Put 3 to 5 drops of the stock blend into a dispersing agent of your choice, such as full-fat powdered or liquid milk (coconut milk is a lovely option) or honey, or directly into the bath salts.

Tip: Always put your essential oils into the dispersing agent first and then stir the mixture around in the bath water as you get into the bath. Spend 15 to 20 minutes soaking in the tub.

ALTERNATE ESSENTIAL OILS: Black Spruce (*Picea mariana*), Rose Geranium (*Pelargonium graveolens* var. *roseum*), and Lavender (*Lavandula angustifolia*)

NOTE: As conifers readily oxidize, use this blend up well within a year. Ideally, take two to three baths per week so the stock blend may be used up within three months.

⇥ Sore Muscle Body Scrub

AUTHOR: Elisabeth Vlasic

Fresh and uplifting, this easy-to-make at home Sore Muscle Body Scrub is indicated for relieving pain while acting as an aid to reducing inflammation in the body. It enlists seven powerful, naturally derived allies known for their anti-inflammatory benefits: rosemary ct. cineole, plai, and wintergreen essential oils, as well as coffee, lavender flowers, magnesium sulfate, and jojoba. The essential oils also offer additional pain-relieving benefits. Furthermore, this scrub exfoliates while softening the skin and helps to hold moisture in the body.

Prep Time: 25 minutes
Yield: Approximately 2 ounces (60 ml)
Safety: Wintergreen should be avoided if one is on anticoagulation medicines. It should also be avoided with children, and if pregnant or breastfeeding. Feel free to use an alternate essential oil if concerned.

INGREDIENTS
- 76 drops Rosemary ct. cineole (*Rosmarinus officinalis*) essential oil
- 41 drops Plai (*Zingiber cassumunar*) essential oil
- 3 drops Nepalese Wintergreen (*Gaultheria fragrantissima*) essential oil
- 1¾ ounces (50 g) fine Epson salt (magnesium sulfate)
- ¼ ounce (7 g) discarded organic coffee beans
- 2 teaspoons (10 g) blended dried lavender flowers
- 2 tablespoons (30 ml) or more Jojoba oil (*Simmondsia chinensis*)

WHAT YOU NEED
- 3 small glass or stainless-steel bowls
- Glass, stainless steel, or wooden stirrer or spoon
- Small scale to weight out coffee and Epsom salt (magnesium sulfate)
- Measuring spoon
- 2-ounce (60 ml) glass jar with lid
- Label

PROCEDURE
1. Measure rosemary, plai, and wintergreen essential oils into a bowl.

2. Gently stir, ensuring the essential oils mix together well. Set aside.

3. In a separate small bowl, mix coffee, Epsom salt, and dried lavender flowers together. Set aside.

4. Add the jojoba to the essential blend.

5. Slowly, in small amounts, add the essential oils blend to the dry ingredients, stirring well to ensure everything is incorporated and it reaches a consistency you like.

6. Spoon into the jar, cap tightly, and label.

How to Use Sore Muscle Body Scrub in Shower: Before you turn the shower on, place a small amount of scrub into your hands, massaging it into your sore muscles in a circular motion to stimulate blood circulation. Once finished, turn the water on and bathe as normal.

NOTE: This is not intended for the delicate facial area.

ALTERNATE ESSENTIAL OILS: Black Pepper (*Piper nigrum*), Helichrysum (*Helichrysum italicum*), and Ginger (*Zingiber officinale*)

NOTE: The essential oil blend in this recipe is created on a 10 percent dilution, which is advised for muscular aches and pains. This works out to 120 drops of essential oil synergy.

✈ Foot Bath Salts to Relieve Swollen Feet

AUTHOR: Amandine Peter

Cold foot baths with Epsom salts are known to help reduce swelling, restore a healthy circulation, and induce relaxation. Essential oils offer various added benefits: Yarrow is naturally astringent and contains a high amount of chamazulene, a potent anti-inflammatory. The cooling/warming effect of peppermint enhances circulation. And cypress relieves fluid accumulation and reduces swelling.

This is a quick and easy recipe to follow. All you have to do is sit down and enjoy!

Prep Time: 5 minutes
Yield: Approximately 4 ounces (115 g)
Safety: Yarrow should be avoided by people taking drugs metabolized by the enzyme CYP1A2. Peppermint should not be used if there are cuts on the skin, or if there is sensitive skin, and should be avoided by all routes if there is cardiac fibrillation or a G6PD deficiency.

INGREDIENTS

- ½ cup (100 g) Epsom salt
- 1 tablespoon (15 ml) Jojoba oil
- 3 drops Yarrow (*Achillea millefolium*) essential oil
- 1 drop Peppermint (*Mentha piperita*) essential oil
- 5 drops Cypress (*Cupressus sempervirens*) essential oil

WHAT YOU NEED

- Small glass or stainless steel bowl
- Glass, stainless steel, or wooden stirrer
- Measuring cups and spoons
- Foot bath basin or bucket

PROCEDURE

1. Place Epsom salt and jojoba oil and in the bowl.

2. Gently stir together for about 30 seconds, ensuring the salt and the oil are fully incorporated.

3. Add essential oils and mix well.

How to Use Foot Bath Salts: Fill the foot bath basin or bucket with cool water. Pour the mix into the water. Sit down and let your feet soak for 15 to 20 minutes.

ALTERNATIVE ESSENTIAL OILS:

Yarrow: German Chamomile (*Matricaria chamomilla* (syn. *Matricaria recutita*) or Roman Chamomile (*Chamaemelum nobile*)
Peppermint: Juniper Berry (*Juniperus communis*) or Helichrysum (*Helichrysum italicum*)
Cypress: Patchouli (*Pogostemon cablin*) or Grapefruit (*Citrus × paradisi*)

⇥ Varicose Vein Aid Gel

AUTHOR: Elisabeth Vlasic

Poor circulation due to damage of or weakness in the walls of veins can cause varicose veins to protrude from the skin. This condition is unsightly and is often painful; it generally occurs on the surface area of the legs. Lack of exercise in one's day-to-day life, constant leg crossing, heredity factors, constipation, pregnancy, being overweight, and poor diet can all contribute to this condition. But don't despair! Certain essential oils, such as rose and cypress, can be highly beneficial by reducing dilation and toning the blood vessels. As the main component of the gel, aloe vera is also a popular remedy for varicose veins due to its wonderful healing, soothing, and protective attributes.

Prep Time: 20 minutes
Yield: Approximately 2 ounces (60 ml)
Shelf Life: Store gel in the refrigerator and use within 3 weeks
Safety: No concerns

INGREDIENTS
- 2 drops Rose (*Rosa × damascena*) essential oil
- 39 drops Cypress (*Cupressus sempervirens*) essential oil
- 29 drops Juniper (*Juniperus communis*) essential oil
- 2 drops Spearmint (*Mentha spicata*) essential oil
- 18 drops Yarrow (*Achillea millefolium*) essential oil
- 2 ounces (57 ml) store-bought aloe vera gel

WHAT YOU NEED
- Small funnel
- Small glass beaker or stainless steel or glass bowl
- Glass, stainless steel, or wooden stirrer or spoon
- 2-ounce (60 ml) flip top squeezy bottle
- Funnel
- Label

PROCEDURE
1. Combine rose, cypress, juniper, spearmint, and yarrow essential oils into the glass beaker.

2. Gently stir, ensuring the essential oils have mixed together well.

3. Add aloe vera gel to the essential oil mixture and stir well.

4. Pour gel into squeezy bottle using a funnel.

5. Cap tightly and label.

How to Use Varicose Vein Aid Gel: Do not press directly on the varicose veins when applying this lotion. Instead, always apply around the vein (above and below), massaging in an upwards motion.

ALTERNATE ESSENTIAL OILS: Black Pepper (*Piper nigrum*), Rose Geranium (*Pelargonium graveolens* var. *roseum*), and Niaouli (*Melaleuca quinquenervia*)

NOTE: This is blended at a 5 percent dilution, which is highlighted for use in a localized remedy; it comes out to 90 drops of essential oil in a 2-ounce (60 ml) product.

When shopping for store-bought aloe vera gel, we suggest always checking the ingredient label to make sure that the product is high-quality, organic, and preferably 100 percent aloe vera gel, thus avoiding the preservatives and additives that some brands add. Feel free to check out our resource list in this book for further guidance.

➵ Diffuser Blend for Hay Fever

AUTHOR: Elisabeth Vlasic

Hay fever, or allergic rhinitis, is an irritating condition that exhibits similar symptoms to the typical cold. However, unlike the common cold, the symptoms are not caused by a viral or bacterial infection, but airborne pollen or other allergens such as cat dander. One may experience an individualized combination of a runny, inflamed, and itchy nose, tingling and swollen eyes, headaches, sneezing, sinus pressure, and congestion.

Hay fever is a tricky ailment to target, as symptoms vary from person-to-person and over-the-counter medicines do not necessarily conquer all that one is exhibiting. For example, antihistamines are responsible for minimizing sneezing and itchiness, as well as drying up the nose, but do not help with sinus pressure. Because of this, you may have to adapt a trial-and-error frame of mind until you figure out what works best for you.

Energetically, this is an expansive and protective diffuser blend recipe that combines a variety of therapeutics to broadly alleviate the symptoms of hay fever. Essential oils are multifactorial, meaning one essential oil can do many things. For example, niaouli, green myrtle, and blue tansy act as antihistamines. At the same time, niaouli, green myrtle, blue tansy, and goldenrod are considered anti-allergenic, while myrtle and niaouli bring their softening balsamic effects to the anti-inflammatory ailments of myrtle and goldenrod.

Prep Time: 15 minutes
Yield: 0.17 ounce (5 ml)
Safety: Niaouli should be avoided around the faces of small children due to its cineole content. Make sure the area is well ventilated and there are intermittent breaks from the diffusion.

INGREDIENTS

- 9 drops Inula (*Dittrichia graveolens* syn. *Inula graveolens*) essential oil
- 23 drops Goldenrod (*Solidago canadensis*) essential oil
- 19 drops Blue Tansy (*Tanacetum annuum*) essential oil
- 15 drops Niaouli ct. cineole (*Melaleuca quinquenervia*) essential oil
- 4 drops Green Myrtle (*Myrtus communis*) essential oil

WHAT YOU NEED

- Small glass or stainless-steel bowl
- Glass, stainless steel or wooden stirrer
- 5 milliliter empty dark-colored bottle with orifice reducer
- Plastic or glass pipette
- Label

PROCEDURE

1. Combine inula, goldenrod, blue tansy, niaouli, and green myrtle essential oils in the bowl.

2. Gently stir together, ensuring the essential oils mix together well.

3. Using a pipette, fill the bottle with the blend.

4. Add orifice reducer, cap tightly, and label.

How to Use Diffuser Blend for Hay Fever:
Following the diffuser manufacturer's instructions, add diffuser blend. Run your diffuser close by when you have hay fever symptoms. If you do not have a diffuser, you can place a few drops of the blend on a tissue and hold it to your nose to breathe in, or to an inside corner of your clothing to diffuse the aroma that way. You can also use a few drops of this blend diluted in a carrier in the bath. Or, add some of the blend into a carrier such as jojoba to place on your hands or chest and inhale it this way.

ALTERNATE ESSENTIAL OILS: Juniper (*Juniperus communis*), German Chamomile (*Matricaria chamomilla* (syn. *Matricaria recutita*), and Ammi/Khella (*Ammi visnaga*)

NOTE: Drop sizes will vary; 77 to 120 drops will fill a 0.17-ounce (5 ml) bottle. Thus, this recipe is an estimate to fill your 5 ml bottle. You can always add or decrease the individual drops as you deem fit for your personal use.

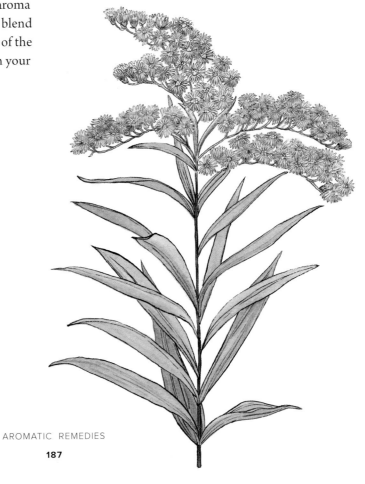

CHAPTER TEN

BLENDING BEYOND RECIPES

WITH SO MANY RECIPES swirling around the World Wide Web through social media, it can be a bit overwhelming to try to tell which ones will really work for you—and expensive to experiment to find out! The answer to this conundrum: to learn how to create and make your own aromatherapy products, be they for your body or your health and wellness. So, where does one begin?

The first questions to ask are:

1. What do you want to make?

2. What is your goal (or goals)?

Once you know the above, you can begin the formulation process. Before diving into how to select your essential oils, though, it is important to distinguish between formulating a body care product versus formulating a synergy. Let's do a quick review of the difference.

A body care product is a combination of essential oils and some type of base, such as a carrier oil and/or herbal oil, an unscented cream or lotion, or a gel or salve. Body care products are designed to be applied to the skin either for the skin or other relevant systems of the body.

A synergy is a combination of essential oils without a carrier/herbal oil or other base. Synergies are designed to be used in diffusers (all types), in personal inhalers, or for steam inhalations.

THE SYNERGY STOCK BOTTLE

You can also make up a synergy called a *stock bottle*. The stock bottle is typically made in ½ to 2 fluid ounce (15 to 60 ml) quantities and is designed to be used over a variety of different methods of application. For instance, let's say it's winter and the cold and flu are going around. You could make up a batch (e.g., 15 ml) of a respiratory synergy with eucalyptus, rosemary, and peppermint. This synergy could then be used in a salve, a chest oil, a diffuser, and even a salt scrub. For each product designed to be used with that specific synergy, you simply add in the desired number of drops based upon your chosen dilution rate.

Below is an overview of the steps you will take depending on whether you are creating a body care product or a synergy.

HOW MUCH IS IN A MILLILITER (ML)?

1 ml = approximately 25 to 35 drops total of essential oil.

HOW TO FORMULATE A BODY CARE PRODUCT

To begin formulating a body care product, you should be able to fill in the following information.

1. **What product are you making?** A body butter, facial oil, or salve, for example.

2. **What is the goal of the product?** To make a beautiful aromatic product? To make a therapeutic product for the skin? To create a synergy for supporting the respiratory system? Something else?

3. **Next, what ingredients make up the product?** Body care products contain a few other ingredients you will need to select when making your product. Here is the table of possible ingredients from chapter 6: Expanding Your Apothecary.

4. **How much are you making?** Decide on the amount.

5. **What is the best dilution rate for your product?** Refer to chart on page 190, Dilution Rate and Indications. Typically, when making a body care product, your dilution will be between 1 and 2.5 percent.

HOW TO FORMULATE A SYNERGY FOR A DIFFUSER OR INHALATION

To begin formulating a synergy for a diffuser or inhalation, you should be able to fill in the following information.

1. **What is the goal for the synergy?** e.g., "uplifting yet calming to stress synergy" or "citrusy."

2. **Synergy ingredients:** Essential oils only.

3. **Decide on the amount you will be making:** e.g., 5- and 10-ml size bottles are two standard sizes for making a small batch of synergy.

BODY CARE PRODUCTS				
	CO	HO	HY	WX
Body and Facial Oils	X	X		
Roll-On (aka Roller Balls)	X	X		
Body Butters	X	X		
Aromatic Gels	X	X	X	
Salves	X	X		X
Lip Balm	X	X		X
Salt Scrubs	X	X		
Unscented Cleansers			X	
Unscented Creams and Lotions	X	X	X	

Key to codes:

CO Carrier oils (includes vegetable oils and specialty seed oils, e.g. rosehip seed, borage, etc.)

HO Herbal oils (e.g. Calendula, St. John's wort, Arnica, etc.)

HY Hydrosol/s

WX Wax

Here is a great reference chart to guide you with dilutions.

DILUTION RATE AND INDICATIONS	
DILUTION IN %	**PURPOSE AND INDICATIONS**
0	Essential oils should not be used for infants under 6 months of age unless absolutely necessary and only if one is trained to do so. Use hydrosols instead.
0.25% to 0.5%	Infants 6 months or older, frail or elderly individuals, immune compromised individuals.
1%	Children 2 to 5 years old.
1.5%	Subtle aromatherapy, emotional and energetic work, facial creams and lotions, exfoliants. Pregnant, frail, or elderly individuals.
2% to 5%	Action on the nervous system, emotional well-being, and response to daily stress. Holistic aromatherapy, general massage work, general skincare, massage oils, lotions, facial oils, body oils, and body butters.
7%	Treatment massage and localized treatment work, wound healing, body oils, butters, and salves.
10%	Muscular aches and pains, trauma injury, treatment massage, acute physical pain, localized treatment work, and salves.
Undiluted	Acute trauma. Use non-aggressive essential oils only.

And once you have your dilution rate chosen, you can figure out your drops using this chart.

ESSENTIAL OIL DILUTION						
Carrier oil	**0.5%**	**1%**	**2.5%**	**3%**	**5%**	**10%**
½ ounce (15 ml)	1–3 drops	3–5 drops	8–11 drops	9–13 drops	15–23 drops	30–46 drops
1 ounce (30 ml)	3–5 drops	6–9 drops	15–23 drops	18–27 drops	30–45 drops	60–90 drops
2 ounces (60 ml)	6–10 drops	12–18 drops	30–46 drops	36–54 drops	60–90 drops	120–180 drops
4 ounces (118 ml)	12–20 drops	24–36 drops	60–92 drops	72–108 drops	120–180 drops	240–360 drops

Formulating Example

1. **Product making:** Facial oil

2. **Goal of product:** To have a beautiful aroma while nourishing the skin and supporting healthy cellular rejuvenation.

3. **Ingredients needed:** Facial oil = carrier/herbal oil(s) + essential oils

4. **Quantity to be made:** 2 fluid ounces (60 ml)

5. **Dilution rate for facial oil:** 1.5 percent, which equals a total of 18 to 27 drops. This is divided among the essential oils you choose to put into the formulation.

Based upon the table above, a 1.5 percent dilution in 2 fluid ounces (60 ml) of carrier would total 48 to 72 drops of essential oil. That's a pretty big range in the number of drops, right? The drops are technically based upon the average number of drops that come out of a typical orifice reducer (the top that allows drops to come out). However, the drop size can vary not only with the same dropper cap but also the different types of orifice reducers used by the variety of essential oil companies. So where does one begin with the number of drops?

At this stage of your learning, it depends on the strength and character, so to speak, of the essential oils you are selecting. If you are blending with heavier essential oils such as rose or vetiver, you could begin on the lower side. If you are blending with lighter or medium strength essential oils, you can move into the higher side. Always leave room to add additional drops. It is far easier to add more essential oil than it is to take them away once they are in the product.

HOW TO SELECT ESSENTIAL OILS

Choosing three to five essential oils to work with requires a bit of practice. Once you have chosen how you are going to approach selecting them, you can then refer to the appropriate charts provided in this chapter to begin narrowing down your selection.

In our blending method, each essential oil we select serves a purpose toward the whole. We select our essential oils with the following approach:

- **The core essential oil.** This is the first essential oil selected. The core essential oil is chosen based upon your primary purpose or goal and is considered the heart of the synergy.

- **The enhancer essential oil.** The enhancer essential oil strengthens the core essential oil in its purpose and therapeutic action.

- **The harmonizer essential oil.** The harmonizing essential oil supports and enhances the vitality and purpose of the overall synergy. The harmonizing essential oil often has a decisive impact on the overall aroma and is chosen for both its aroma and its ability to enhance the goals of the synergy.

- **Additional essential oils.** Optionally, you can decide to add one or two additional essential oils. This addition could be a core, enhancer, and/or harmonizer essential oil or essential oils. You decide!

Now let's get down to the nitty gritty of selecting your essential oils. There are a few ways to begin this process. On the next few pages are three reference charts that have been designed to assist you in your selection.

These charts consist of:

1. **The Aromatic Palette:** The tables provided in this palette are based upon different aromatic qualities, such as citrusy or forest. The aromatic palette provides a path of selecting essential oils based upon the aromatics desired. Let's say you would like to make an inhaler that is reminiscent of the forest; you could select fir, pine, and cypress from the forest palette. Or you could change the forest-only aroma to one that has a bit of citrus in it. Choose two essential oils from the forest palette and one from the citrus palette.

2. **The Therapeutics Chart:** The therapeutics chart categorizes essential oils based upon their affinities to different systems of the body. If you are seeking to make a respiratory remedy or a remedy that reduces menstrual cramps, this is the chart you will want to use.

3. **Morphology (Plant Part) Chart:** The morphology chart is based upon the energetic messages of the essential oil based upon the part of the plant it is derived from.

If approaching your product with emotions in mind, you may begin your search by using the aromatic palette or the morphology approach. If you are formulating a product or synergy for a health imbalance (e.g., respiratory congestion or sluggish digestion) then you can utilize the therapeutics chart.

Once you have selected the essential oils you would like to use in your product formulation, the next question before blending them together is:

Do they smell good together?

This is always done *before* blending them together. Remove the caps from all three to five bottles, place them together in your hands to ensure that all the bottle neck openings are the same height, and then waft the bottles under your nose.

What you want to notice is if the essential oils smell good together and if they appear to merge into one aroma as a group. If one essential oil seems to not merge very well with the others, you may decide to replace that one with another of similar aroma or therapeutic action. Whether blending for emotional/mental/spiritual or physical benefits, the essential oils should be complementary and supportive to one another in action and aroma.

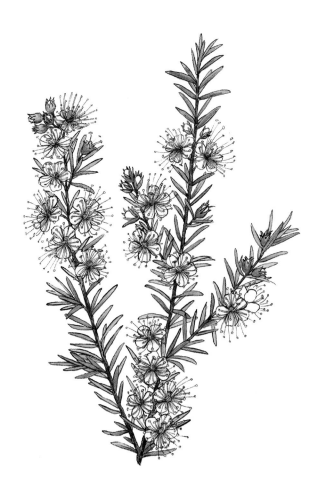

AROMATIC PALETTES

FOREST AROMAS

Essential Oil	Latin name
Cedarwood	*Cedrus deodara*
Cedarwood, Virginia	*Juniperus virginiana*
Cypress	*Cupressus sempervirens*
Fir, Balsam	*Abies balsamea*
Juniper Berry	*Juniperus communis*
Pine, Scots	*Pinus sylvestris*
Pinyon Pine	*Pinus edulis*
Spruce, Hemlock	*Tsuga canadensis*

CITRUS AROMAS

Essential Oil	Latin name
Bergamot	Citrus bergamia
Grapefruit	*Citrus × paradisi*
Lemon	*Citrus limon*
Lime	*Citrus × aurantifolia*
Sweet Orange	*Citrus sinensis*
Mandarin	*Citrus reticulata*

SPICY AROMAS

Essential Oil	Latin name
Black Pepper	*Piper nigrum*

SPICY AROMAS

Essential Oil	Latin name
Cardamom	*Elettaria cardamomum*
Cinnamon Leaf	*Cinnamomum verum* (syn. *Cinnamomum zeylanicum*)
Clove Bud	*Syzygium aromaticum*
Ginger	*Zingiber officinale*
Turmeric	*Curcuma longa*

FLORAL AROMAS

Common Name	Latin name
Geranium	*Pelargonium × asperum*
Jasmine	*Jasminum grandiflorum* (or *Jasminum officinale*)
Lavender	*Lavandula angustifolia*
Neroli	*Citrus aurantium* var. *amara*
Petitgrain	*Citrus aurantium* var. *amara*
Rose	*Rosa × damascena* or *Rosa alba*
Ylang Ylang	*Cananga odorata*

RESIN AROMAS

Essential Oil	Latin name
Frankincense	*Boswellia sacra* (syn. *Boswellia carteri*)
Myrrh	*Commiphora myrrha*

THERAPEUTICS

SYSTEM AFFINITY	THERAPEUTICS
Circulatory (cardiovascular) system	**To support healthy circulation:** Black Pepper, Celery Seed, Juniper Berry, Lemon, Rosemary ct. cineole **Varicose veins**, to improve appearance of or prevent them from getting worse: Cypress, Lemon, Patchouli, Rose
Digestive system	**Relieve nausea:** Ginger, Peppermint **Relieve excess gas:** Anise, Cardamom, Cilantro, Coriander Seed, Sweet Fennel, Ginger, Peppermint **To support and enhance the digestive system (stimulating):** Anise, Black Pepper, Carrot Seed, Celery Seed, Sweet Fennel, Fingerroot, Ginger, Peppermint
Musculoskeletal system	**To relieve pain:** Roman Chamomile, Clary Sage, Clove Bud, Coriander Seed, Ginger, Laurel, Lemongrass, Sweet Marjoram, Peppermint, Plai, Rosemary ct. camphor, Vetiver, Wintergreen **To relieve muscle spasms:** Bergamot Mint, Roman Chamomile, Clary Sage, Coriander Seed, Lavender, Sweet Marjoram **To relieve muscular tension:** Basil ct. linalool, Bergamot Mint, Roman Chamomile, Clary Sage, Coriander Seed, Katafray, Lavender, Sweet Marjoram, Pinyon Pine, Hemlock Spruce, Vetiver To support recovery from sprains, strains, and repetitive injuries, herbal oils such as Arnica and St. John's wort can play a central role with essential oils.
Respiratory system	**Allergies:** to prevent or relieve allergies, use a personal inhaler: Blue Tansy, German Chamomile, Goldenrod **Decongesting and helpful for eliminating excess mucus in the nasal cavity:** Cardamom, Blue Gum Eucalyptus, Fingerroot, Laurel, Green Myrtle, Niaouli, Peppermint, Rosemary ct. cineole, Saro **Immune Supportive Essential Oils:** Frankincense, Laurel, Niaouli, Hemlock Spruce, Lemon, Thyme ct. thymol **Relieve spasmodic cough:** Cardamom, Cypress, Laurel, Saro **Help to clear congestion in lungs:** Anise, Cardamom, Blue Gum Eucalyptus, Fingerroot, Inula, Laurel, Green Myrtle, Rosemary ct. cineole, Saro
Reproductive system	**For painful menstrual cramps or menstrual periods:** Clary Sage, Sweet Fennel, Lavender, Sweet Marjoram, Plai **To uplift during challenging times, mood swings, or mild depression:** Bergamot, Clary Sage, Neroli, Sweet Orange, Patchouli, Petitgrain, Mandarin, Rose, Ylang Ylang **To increase sexual desire/aphrodisiacs:** Cardamom, Cinnamon Leaf, Clary Sage, Ginger, Jasmine Absolute, Patchouli, Rose, Ylang Ylang **To support hormonal balance:** Clary Sage, Geranium, Lavender

EMOTIONS

In this emotion-based blending method, we are using the information contained in the plant part to send an energetic message via its aroma. Also called Morphology, this method was developed by Jade Shutes early on in her aromatherapy career and was first published in her *Blending Manual* in 1992. Other aromatherapy educators and books have since shared this approach to blending and selecting essential oils.

Blending by Morphology approaches the client and the essential oils based upon the unique message that each individual oil contains, based upon the part of the plant which they are obtained from. In the following pages you will uncover the messages that seeds, roots, woods, resins, leaves, needles, fruits, and flowers have to impart.

SEEDS

Seeds represent the beginning of life for a plant, its potential to become and to manifest. Seed essential oils naturally have an affinity for the reproductive system. They can support growth and manifestation, new beginnings, embarking upon a journey, and restorative work on the self.

ROOTS

One of the functions of a root is to anchor the plant into a substrate (such as the soil). Root essential oils contain messages to ground, provide stability, nourish and support, and maintain homeostasis (a balance in the body). They provide strength and stability.

WOOD

The wood (trunk) is the center and strength of a tree. Therefore on an emotional level, essential oils that come from the wood can provide strength and centeredness. They encourage the individual to go inward and inspire self-reflection. For example, if things are scattered or overwhelming, wood essen-

tial oils help facilitate going within our center and reflecting on what is happening.

RESINS

If you cut into certain trees, they release a resinous substance that helps to protect and heal the tree. Resin essential oils therefore contain the inherent energy to protect and to heal. Resin energy is about healing and is particularly indicated for emotional wounding such as trauma, heartbreak, grieving, and separation. It is powerful when used during meditation practice to reconnect with the divine or one's spirituality.

LEAVES AND NEEDLES

Leaves and needles have a natural affinity for the respiratory system and hence are connected to the breath and breathing. They inspire deep, expansive breathing that can lend itself to feelings of empowerment and vitality.

Leaves and needles function within plants for photosynthesis. If we consider photosynthesis for a moment, we can see that this is connected to the power of transformation. Leaf and needle essential oils allow for shifting in perceptions or states of being that may not be productive to an individual's life.

FLOWERS

Flowers have a strong affinity with the emotional realm and offer a more feminine energy. Since antiquity, they have represented something of beauty, relating to love and a gift of friendship, hence their ability to soothe the heart and mind. Flowers therefore have a relationship with the reproductive system, our ability to attract, and our ability to survive difficulties. The flower inspires another generation of growth and gives forth life, potential, and movement forward.

Essential oils made from flowers are encoded with messages representing love, compassion, forgiveness, emotional nourishment, attraction, creation, manifestation, and beauty.

FRUIT

Citrus fruits have a naturally uplifting and cleansing effect. Fruits contain the message of purification—cleansing and releasing that which binds or prevents one from moving forward. They are incredibly beneficial for those who feel "heavy" energetically,

that is, stuck or unable to release certain thoughts and/or feelings. Citrus oils can also relieve anxiety. When used with roots and resins, they can be quite stabilizing while clarifying difficult situations or allowing for movement of challenging emotions.

Now that we understand the potential message an essential oil may impart based upon the part of the plant it is extracted from, the chart below provides indications and examples of essential oils covered in this book for each category.

PART OF PLANT	INDICATED FOR	ESSENTIAL OILS
Seeds	Inability to manifest, frustration, lack of communication between two people, inability to digest one's food and/or to gain nourishment, exhaustion, having difficulty conceiving ideas, boredom or inability to be in the present moment, imbalances of the second chakra or the solar plexus chakra, frigidity, hopelessness, cynicism, lack of self-esteem, frustration	Angelica Seed, Cardamom, Carrot Seed, Coriander Seed, Sweet Fennel
Roots	Flightiness, instability, anxiety, feelings of being overwhelmed, scattered, sensitive constitution, nervousness, feelings of being disconnected to life, frazzled nerves, envy, compulsiveness, panic attacks, irritability, worry	Angelica Root, Ginger, Vetiver
Wood	Insecurity, lack of self-esteem, a need to go inward, self-reflection, need to conduct energy either upwards or downwards, weak constitution, envy	Himalayan Cedarwood
Resins	Post-traumatic stress, emotional wounds, anxiety, feelings of frustration, irritability, poor or lack of self-esteem, spiritual void or challenges, recovery from addictions or abuse, psychic wounding, lack of self-love and/or nourishment, impatience, tension, worry, despondency, bitterness, anger, anxiety	Copaiba, Frankincense, Myrrh
Leaves and Needles	Lack of confidence and/or self-esteem issues, shallow breathing, feelings of being hemmed in by life, contracted unable to expand, difficulty expressing emotions, stagnation, unable to shift or change/grow, lack of vitality, lack of **courage**, irritability, tension	Cypress, Basil ct. linalool, Blue Gum Eucalyptus, Balsam Fir, Laurel, Green Myrtle, Niaouli, Petitgrain, Peppermint, Pinyon Pine, Hemlock Spruce

PART OF PLANT	INDICATED FOR	ESSENTIAL OILS
Flowers	Anger, anxiety, burnout, lack of confidence, being critical of others, depression, despondency, lack of empathy, emptiness, frigidity, grief, grumpiness, guilt feelings, hopelessness, hostility, jealousy, insecurity, instability, resentment, resignation, sadness, self-criticism (to bring back into body, inner awareness), self-esteem issues, shyness, stress, tension, inability to forgive	Roman Chamomile, German Chamomile, Clary Sage, Geranium, Helichrysum, Jasmine, Lavender, Neroli, Rose, Yarrow, Ylang Ylang
Fruits	Toxic thinking that turns in on the self, anger, self-criticism, cynicism, mild depression, despondency, frigidity, grief, grumpiness, guilt feelings, hopelessness, hostility, inability to forgive or let go, indecision (when decision is creating anxiety), insecurity, resentment, resignation, sadness, stress, tension	Bergamot, Grapefruit, Lemon, Mandarin, Sweet Orange

Inspire and Warm

For someone who is feeling depressed due to low energy, feels cold, and lacks vitality.

Fruit: 10 drops Sweet Orange to uplift, inspire, and support vitality
Root: 7 drops Ginger for warmth
Flower: 5 drops Neroli for acceptance and kindness to self, inspires
Leaves and Needles: 2 drops Pinyon Pine to support vitality, 1 ounce (30 ml) Sesame oil

Grief Inhaler

Flower: 5 drops Rose for nourishing the heart and compassion
Fruit: 10 drops Tangerine to warm and comfort while also gently uplifting; a beam of sunshine
Root: 3 drops Vetiver to connect with and ground the grieving process
Resin: 5 drops Frankincense for healing and protection

SYSTEM AFFINITY REVIEW

BODY SYSTEM AND ESSENTIAL OILS

Circulatory
Black Pepper
Celery Seed
Cypress
Juniper Berry
Lemon
Rose
Rosemary ct. cineole

Reproductive
Basil ct. linalool
Clary Sage
Sweet Fennel
Geranium
Jasmine Absolute
Lavender
Mandarin
Sweet Marjoram
Neroli
Petitgrain
Plai
Rose

Respiratory
Anise
Blue Tansy
Cardamom
Cinnamon Leaf
Cypress
Eucalyptus Globulus
Fingerroot
Balsam Fir
Goldenrod
Inula
Laurel
Sweet Marjoram
Green Myrtle
Niaouli
Peppermint
Scots Pine
Pinyon Pine
Plai
Rosemary ct. cineole
Rosemary ct. camphor
Saro
Hemlock Spruce
Thyme ct. thymol

Skin
Calendula CO_2
Cape Chamomile
Carrot Seed
Himalayan Cedarwood
German Chamomile
Roman Chamomile
Cistus
Copaiba
Cypress
Frankincense
Geranium
Helichrysum
Lavender
Melissa
Neroli
Niaouli
Palmarosa
Patchouli
Petitgrain
Rose
Rosemary ct. verbenone
Blue Tansy
Thyme ct. linalool
Yarrow

Digestive
Angelica Root
Anise
Basil ct. linalool
Bergamot
Black Pepper
Cardamom
Carrot Seed
Celery Seed
German Chamomile
Roman Chamomile
Cilantro
Cinnamon Leaf
Coriander Seed
Sweet Fennel
Fingerroot
Ginger
Grapefruit
Lemon
Mandarin
Sweet Orange
Peppermint
Thyme ct. thymol
Thyme ct. linalool

Musculoskeletal
Basil ct. linalool
Bergamot Mint
Black Pepper
Himalayan Cedarwood
Roman Chamomile
Clary Sage
Clove Bud
Coriander Seed
Ginger
Juniper Berry
Katafray
Laurel
Lavender
Lemongrass
Sweet Marjoram
Peppermint
Plai
Pinyon Pine
Rosemary ct. cineole or
Rosemary ct. camphor
Hemlock Spruce
Vetiver
Wintergreen

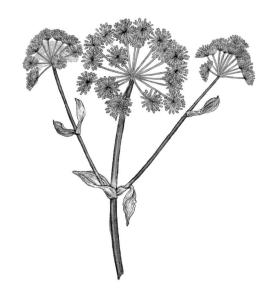

RESOURCES

We hope this book has inspired you to learn more about plants and essential oils. Perhaps you will start building your own collection of essential oils and botanical ingredients to have easily on-hand. Or perhaps this book motivated you to make a change and become a Certified Aromatherapist, weaving your discoveries and experiences with the oils into a new career.

Whatever path you are on, whether you are considering a more professional route or are interested in caring for your immediate family and friends, these tips and recommendations will support your journey. We've organized our favorite resources all in one place.

LET'S START WITH THE ESSENTIAL OILS

Everyone always asks us what brands of essential oils we like. And to be honest, we avoid focusing our attention on just one brand. For us, the first and most important relationship is with the plant and how it smells. In other words, we recommend suspending your attachment to any one brand and instead pay attention to how your experience with the essential oil and the plant affects your body and your mind. That means our main focus is on cultivating a relationship with authentic and genuine essential oils that can easily be traced from seed to the still.

Now that you've read our book, you understand how vital it is to cultivate a full sensory experience with plants. By exercising our sense of smell, by observing the plants as they grow and move through different seasons and environments, and by also touching and tasting them, we can open our hearts and our minds to a much deeper understanding of their physical and energetic properties.

This is why it is so important for us to share several different sources with our students and our community. By doing so, we are inviting you to take responsibility for knowing the oils on your own terms, to develop and expand your own olfactory palate, and to connect to the plant and oil in ways that echo far beyond the molecules that compose them.

We have spent many years, a combined total of more than 50, smelling oils from many different countries, brands, distilleries, suppliers, and distributors. This is our treasured list of sources that we trust 100 percent.

ABOUT ACCREDITATION AND LICENSING

It's apparent that essential oils are here to stay! The practice of using them, whether at home or professionally, requires that the education we receive is from a trusted source. And you may want the confidence and assurance of having professional credentials that recognize the time you've spent learning and practicing.

For those of you wondering what it means to be a Certified Aromatherapist, let's clarify some terminology regarding certification and licensing.

As a practice, aromatherapy is not a licensed or regulated profession in the United States. And that's not a bad thing! Rather than licensing, the industry is guided by professional organizations such as National Association for Holistic Aromatherapists (NAHA) in the United States, and other professional aromatherapy organizations throughout the world. These organizations set education and professional standards for aromatherapy schools to voluntarily comply with.

Professional aromatherapy organizations like the NAHA, do not certify aromatherapists. Certification is provided by individual schools based upon specific criteria for each level of aromatherapy training as approved by the respective organizations.

Certification is earned from the school you choose to attend, which is why selecting a balanced, progressive, and inspiring school is so valuable.

Whether you are adding aromatherapy to an existing profession or are part of the 21st century wellness movement, becoming a Certified Aromatherapist means you will be recognized as having acquired the knowledge, skills, and tools that not only comply with industry and professional standards but support your success as part of the new generation of aromatherapists.

ESSENTIAL OIL SUPPLIERS

AMRITA
www.amrita.net

EDEN BOTANICALS
www.edenbotanicals.com

ENFLEURAGE: AROMATICS FROM THE NATURAL WORLD www.enfleurage.com

FLORIHANA
www.florihana.com/en/

NATURE'S GIFT
www.naturesgift.com

ORIGINAL SWISS AROMATICS
www.originalswissaromatics.com

PHIBEE AROMATICS
www.phibeearomatics.com

PRANAROM
www.pranarom.com

ZAYAT AROMA
www.zayataroma.com

CERTIFIED ORGANIC BOTANICAL INGREDIENTS

Includes butters, waxes, salts, herbs, powders, carrier oils, herbal infused oils, and antioxidants.

BANYAN BOTANICALS
www.banyanbotanicals.com

BOTANICAL INNOVATIONS
www.botanicinnovations.com

FROM NATURE WITH LOVE
www.fromnaturewithlove.com

JEDWARDS INTERNATIONAL, INC.
(bulk natural oils) www.bulknaturaloils.com

THE JOJOBA COMPANY
www.jojobacompany.com

MOUNTAIN ROSE HERBS
www.mountainroseherbs.com

OH, OH ORGANICS
www.ohohorganic.com

PACIFIC BOTANICALS
www.pacificbotanicals.com

STARWEST BOTANICALS
www.starwest-botanicals.com/category/bulk-herbs

HYDROSOLS

EDEN BOTANICALS
www.edenbotanicals.com

MORNING MYST BOTANICALS
www.morningmystbotanics.com

PHIBEE AROMATICS
www.phibeearomatics.com

PRANAROM
www.pranarom.com

OUR FAVORITE AROMATHERAPY AUTHORS

Salvatore Battaglia
Dominique Baudoux
Jane Buckle
Nicholas Culpeper
Ann Harman
Peter Holmes
Julia Lawless
Gabriel Mojay
Jennifer Peace Rhind
Shirley Price
Jeanne Rose
Kurt Schnaubelt
Robert Tisserand
Valerie Ann Worwood

CONTAINERS, BOTTLES, JARS, AND LABELS

CONTAINER AND PACKAGING
www.containerandpackaging.com

INFINITY JARS
www.infinityjars.com

ONLINE LABELS
www.onlinelabels.com

PREMIUM VIALS
www.premiumvials.com

SKS BOTTLE & PACKAGING
www.sks-bottle.com

SPECIALTY BOTTLE
www.specialtybottle.com

PROFESSIONAL ASSOCIATIONS

AMERICAN BOTANICAL COUNCIL
www.abc.herbalgram.org

AMERICAN HERBALISTS GUILD
www.americanherbalistsguild.com

CANADIAN FEDERATION OF AROMATHERAPISTS
www.cfacanada.com

INTERNATIONAL FEDERATION OF PROFESSIONAL AROMATHERAPISTS www.ifparoma.org

NATIONAL ASSOCIATION OF HOLISTIC AROMATHERAPY www.naha.org

ONLINE RESEARCH AND RESOURCES

AMERICAN BOTANICAL COUNCIL
www.abc.herbalgram.org

AMERICAN HERBALISTS GUILD
www.americanherbalistsguild.com

A MODERN HERBAL
www.botanical.com/botanical/mgmh/mgmh.html

AROMA WEB
www.aromaweb.com

INTERNATIONAL JOURNAL OF CLINICAL AROMATHERAPY www.ijca.net

INTERNATIONAL JOURNAL OF PROFESSIONAL HOLISTIC AROMATHERAPY www.ijpha.com

PUBMED
https://pubmed.ncbi.nlm.nih.gov

ABOUT THE AUTHORS

JADE SHUTES, B.A., Dipl. AT, Cert. Herbalist, has been practicing and studying forms of natural healing for nearly three decades. She was one of the vanguard of professionals who helped introduce aromatherapy to the US in the early 1990s. A prolific writer, Jade has influenced a generation of aromatherapy practitioners and home users with her balanced and progressive approach to the use of essential oils. She is the former President of National Association for Holistic Aromatherapy (NAHA). Her course Aromatic Medicine was a landmark course providing worldwide education on the internal use of essential oils.

An aromatherapy educator for over thirty years, Jade opened one of the first aromatherapy schools in United States. Jade spends much of her time in the Appalachia mountains of Virginia growing and distilling aromatic plants on her land, offering retreats, and expanding her relationship with the land and her community.

AMY GALPER, B.A., M.A., has been a certified aromatherapist since 2001, as well as a passionate advocate, entrepreneur, formulator, and consultant in clean beauty and wellness. She is the co-author of *Plant Powered Beauty* and endorsed by beauty industry visionary Bobbi Brown, Credo Beauty's Annie Jackson, Sophie Uliano, and Tata Harper. Amy is a member of Credo Beauty's Clean Beauty Council, celebrating, advocating and educating for Clean Beauty and Wellness, along with other influencers and thought leaders in the field.

She is a guest lecturer at New York University and has presented at Nova Southeastern University (NSU). She has been featured on Fox News, Thrive, Reuters, and has been quoted as an aromatherapy expert for countless print articles, television, podcasts, and online posts.

CONTRIBUTORS

AMY ANTHONY is a certified clinical aromatherapist, certified Aromatic Studies Method teacher, herbalist, gardener, and artisanal distiller with a private aromatherapy practice based in Manhattan. She is a graduate of the New York Institute of Aromatherapy where she earned her level 1 and level 2 aromatherapy certifications and is registered with the National Association for Holistic Aromatherapy. Read more of Amy's writing and about her practice at https://nycaroma.com.

AMANDINE PETER graduated from the New York Institute of Aromatic Studies, and eventually became a certified clinical aromatherapist and a certified Aromatic Studies Method teacher. In 2017, following her desire to harmonize aromatherapy with other healing modalities, she became a reiki master. She also teaches aromatherapy and herbalism classes at the New York Botanical Garden since 2018.

ELISABETH VLASIC, please call her Libby, is a certified aromatherapist and essential oil educator. She is a certified herbalist having attended Arbor Vitae School of Traditional Herbalism in New York City. A dedicated forever student of the plant-world, Libby was honored to be a senior teacher at the New York Institute of Aromatic Studies for many years.

ACKNOWLEDGMENTS

To Jan Kusmirek, for inspiring me to think outside the box of traditional aromatherapy and to my son, Soren, for his love and support.

—JS

I could not have written this book without the love and support from my husband, my parents, my mother-in-law, my sisters-in-law, my brother-in-law, my nephews, and my entire extended family. I also want to deeply thank all the students who passed through the doors of my school, The New York Institute of Aromatherapy, and the gifted team of teachers, Amy Anthony, Amandine Pete,r and Elisabeth Vlasic, whose recipes are shared within the chapters of this book. A special thanks is also due to Celeste Knopf, who continues to make sure our work is accessible and shared. A huge shout out to Jill Alexander, our editor, who shepherded this book to manifest—along with the whole team at Fair Winds Press who made this possible. Baruch Hashem!

—AG

ENDNOTES

1. Shutes, J. (2000). Foundations of Aromatherapy certificate coursebook. New York Institute of Aromatic Studies.

2. IBID

3. Holmes, P. (2016). *Aromatica: A Clinical Guide to Essential Oil Therapeutics*. Volume 1: Principles and Profiles, Philadelphia, PA: Singing Dragon.

4. IBID

5. Tisserand, R. and Young, R. (2014) *Essential Oil Safety*, 2nd Edition. Milton, ON, CA: Churchill Livingstone Elsevier.

6. https://www.ewg.org/news/news-releases/2007/02/08/ewg-research-shows-22-percent-all-cosmetics-may-be-contaminated-cancer. The EWG is a non-profit, non-partisan organization dedicated to protecting human health and the environment. They cover issues and research from ingredients in body care products to what pesticides might appear in the food we are eating.

7. Throughout this book, we cover aromatherapy and essential oil content relevant to applying essential oils to the skin and via inhalation or diffusion (olfaction and respiratory system). Although we believe in the efficacy of utilizing essential oils internally, that topic is not covered in this book. We believe one needs further education than what we could share in a book of this nature and length.

8. Sense of Smell Institute, Ltd. (1992). *Living Well with Your Sense of Smell*. New York, N.Y.

9. Wilson, D. and Stevenson, R. (2006). *Learning to Smell: Olfactory Perception from Neurobiology to Behavior*. Baltimore, MD: John Hopkins University Press.

10. Mills, S. and Bone K., (2012). *Principles and Practice of Phytotherapy: Modern Herbal Medicine*. Milton, ON, CA: Churchill Livingstone Elsevier.

11. IBID

12. Schnaubelt, K. (2011). *The Healing Intelligence of Essential Oils: The Science of Advanced Aromatherapy*. Rochester, VT: Healing Arts Press.

INDEX

H

hay fever: Diffuser Blend for Hay Fever, 186–187

health
definition of, 12
goals for, 12–13

Helichrysum (*Helichrysum italicum*)
Foot Bath Salts to Relieve Swollen Feet, 184
hydrosol, 157
Sore Muscle Body Scrub, 183
Steam Inhalation for Bronchitis, 175

Hemlock Spruce (*Tsuga canadensis*), 117

herbal oils, 148, 153
arnica, 153
ingredients chart, 148
skin imbalances and, 35–36
St. John's wort, 153

Himalayan Cedarwood (*Cedrus deodara*), 78

Holmes, Peter, 21

hydrosols
Aromatherapy Foaming Cleanser for Hands, 167
Calendula, 156
Clary Sage, 156
German Chamomile, 156
Helichrysum, 157
ingredient chart, 148
Lavender, 157
Neroli, 157
overview, 155–156
Rose, 157
Rose Geranium, 156
skin conditions, 35–36
Witch Hazel, 157

hypertension: Tension Release Spritzer, 42

I

indigestion
Inhaler to Relieve Indigestion, 181
Tummy Massage Oil to Help Prevent Indigestion, 180

inhalation
Grief Inhaler, 197
Inhaler to Relieve Emotional Turmoil from PMS, 173
Inhaler to Relieve Indigestion, 181
personal inhaler tubes, 172
smelling salts, 173
steam inhalation, 174–175
Steam Inhalation for Bronchitis, 175

synergy formulation, 189–191

insomnia: Sleepy Time Diffuser Blend for Insomnia, 41

Inula (*Dittrichia graveolens* syn. *Inula graveolens*)
Diffuser Blend for Hay Fever, 186–187
mini-monograph, 101
Steam Inhalation for Bronchitis, 175

J

Jasmine (*Jasminum grandiflorum*)
mini-monograph, 90
Self-Love Botanical Perfume, 43

Jojoba (*Simmondsia chinensis*)
Calm and Nourish roll-on, 160
Candelilla Lip Balm, 164
Compassion and Strength roll-on, 160
Foot Bath Salts to Relieve Swollen Feet, 184
Forest Blend roll-on, 160
lip balms, 164
overview, 151
Self-Love Botanical Perfume, 43
Sore Muscle Body Scrub, 183
Tummy Massage Oil to Help Prevent Indigestion, 180

Juniper (*Juniperus communis*)
Diffuser Blend for Hay Fever, 186–187
Foot Bath Salts to Relieve Swollen Feet, 184
mini-monograph, 53
Varicose Vein Aid Gel, 185

K

Katafray (*Cedrelopsis grevei*), 83

ketones, 20

Khella/Ammi (*Ammi visnaga*)
Diffuser Blend for Hay Fever, 186–187
mini-monograph, 92
Tension Release Spritzer, 42

L

Laurel (*Laurus nobilis*)
mini-monograph, 87
Steam Inhalation for Bronchitis, 175

Lavender (*Lavandula angustifolia*)
Aromatherapy Foaming Cleanser for Hands, 167
Candelilla Lip Balm, 164
hydrosol, 157

Inhaler to Relieve Emotional Turmoil from PMS, 173
mini-monograph, 129
Natural Hand Protective Gel, 162
Salve for Joint Pain, 178–179
Sleepy Time Diffuser Blend for Insomnia, 41
Soothing Bath Blend for Restless Legs, 182
Sore Muscle Body Scrub, 183
Steam Inhalation for Bronchitis, 175
Tension Release Spritzer, 42
Whipped Body Butter, 161

Lavendin (*Lavandula x intermedia*), 130

Lemon (*Citrus limon*)
mini-monograph, 132
Natural Hand Protective Gel, 162
steam inhalation, 174
Steam Inhalation for Bronchitis, 175

Lemongrass (*Cymbopogon citratus*), 88

lip balm
Candelilla Lip Balm, 164
ingredient chart, 148

lotions, 168

M

Mandarin (*Citrus reticulata*)
Inhaler to Relieve Emotional Turmoil from PMS, 173
Inhaler to Relieve Indigestion, 181
mini-monograph, 70

massage oil: Tummy Massage Oil to Help Prevent Indigestion, 180

Maury, Marguerite, 11–12

May Chang (*Litsea cubeba*), 135

memories, 40

mild essential oils, 21–22

monoterpene alcohols, 19

monoterpenes, 19

Moroccan chamomile. *See* Blue Tansy.

morphology (plant parts), 196–197

musculoskeletal system
affinity review, 198
skin and, 29
therapeutics, 194

Myrrh (*Commiphora myrrha*), 162

N

Natural Hand Protective Gel, 162

nebulizing diffusers, 170

neem oil, 151

Nepalese Wintergreen (*Gaultheria fragrantissima*), 183